A post-graduate's guide to doing a literature review in health and social care

A post-graduate's guide to doing a literature review in health and social care

Helen Aveyard, Sheila Payne and Nancy Preston

Open University Press

Open University Press
McGraw-Hill Education
McGraw-Hill House
Shoppenhangers Road
Maidenhead
Berkshire
England
SL6 2QL

email: enquiries@openup.co.uk
world wide web: www.openup.co.uk

and Two Penn Plaza, New York, NY 10121-2289, USA

First published 2016

A catalogue record of this book is available from the British Library

ISBN-13: 978-0-33-526368-4
ISBN-10: 0-33-526368-2
eISBN: 978-0-33-526369-1

Library of Congress Cataloging-in-Publication Data
CIP data applied for

Typeset by Transforma Pvt. Ltd., Chennai, India

Printed by Bell and Bain Ltd, Glasgow

Fictitious names of companies, products, people, characters and/or data
that may be used herein (in case studies or in examples) are not intended to
represent any real individual, company, product or event.

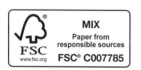

MIX
Paper from
responsible sources

FSC
www.fsc.org   FSC® C007785

Praise for this book

"Consistently clear and concise and using contemporary examples of research applied to the descriptions of methodology, this guide will be useful and accessible at whichever stage in your post-graduate project you come across it. For those people pondering the most suitable approach to literature reviewing to use, it provides answers to fundamental and technical questions. For those already immersed in their chosen approach, the style and layout will make it a refreshing resource. The breadth of content will demystify approaches that are unfamiliar but that are necessary to understand. A highly readable guide whatever your health or social care topic."

Clare Oakland, PhD Student, Department of Primary Care and Population Health, University College London, UK

Contents

Introduction

We have written this book in order to highlight the importance and relevance of the literature review to your post-graduate project; whether your project is a small-scale study or a larger project at PhD or doctoral level – or somewhere in between. At all levels of post-graduate study, you need to engage with an extensive amount of existing literature, in order to justify, inform and develop your project.

As you start to think about your post-graduate studies, you have already begun to read around your topic and you may have encountered a vast selection of literature: for example research, discussion, theories, views and opinions. You may be wondering how to make sense of what you are reading and how you might integrate these different types of evidence into your literature review at the level expected of a post-graduate student.

While this can seem daunting, the aim of this book is to guide you through the types of literature you will encounter and the ways these can be integrated into your post-graduate project. We will also describe the different methods of literature review that can be used and help you to identify the one that is most appropriate for your study. You will see that we refer to a variety of methods for conducting a literature review. It is beyond the scope of this book to discuss all the approaches in detail. If you decide to focus in depth on a particular method, we will refer you to an appropriate text.

Literature reviews are becoming increasingly important in health and social care. This is because there is an increasing amount of published material, which means that it is impossible for any one practitioner to keep up to date with every piece of research in his or her area. A literature review therefore provides a summary of the research and other relevant information on a particular research question to inform practice. A literature review is also an essential pre-requisite prior to any empirical study.

Therefore, different projects need different approaches to literature reviewing. Some projects will use the existing literature to justify a larger empirical research study while others will use the existing literature to answer a question without proceeding on to an empirical study. The methods of doing these literature reviews are the same, but there may be a subtle difference in the emphasis of the review, depending on its role in your project (Figure I.1).

The importance of a rigorous approach to reviewing the literature, rather than simply 'cherry picking' literature that is relevant to your review, prior to an empirical study is increasingly recognized. It is also acknowledged that the literature review can be a study in its own right. The importance of the literature review has been influenced by the emergence of the Cochrane and Campbell Collaborations and their systematic approach to literature reviewing. These collaborations were developed as part of the move towards evidence-based practice, which has challenged practitioners to use the best available evidence to inform their practice. The Cochrane and Campbell Collaborations have drawn attention to the importance of the literature review and as a result, in many areas of health and social care, there are summaries of evidence to guide practice and online access to systematic reviews, which are published through various professional organizations.

The increasing importance of the literature review within health and social care has led to a re-energizing of the role of the literature review

Your literature review is likely to have one
of the following roles in your project

| As a pre-requisite to a subsequent empirical study; the literature review identifies gaps in knowledge and justifies your forthcoming research study. | As a standalone literature review; the literature review is a project in its own right and does not directly lead to an empirical study, although it might indicate that further research is needed. |

Figure I.1 Different uses of the literature in a review

within post-graduate projects; we argue that the literature review should be regarded as a central component of your project and a research project in its own right, which can be written up and submitted for publication. It is worth noting that a literature review that has been undertaken rigorously is more likely to be accepted for publication as a piece of research in its own right.

In this book, we will discuss the underlying principles for doing a literature review in a robust and systematic manner, and these are principles common to all reviews. This includes how to search and make sense of the literature you find. This will be explained in more depth than you may have considered at undergraduate level.

Once you have identified your literature review question(s), your aim is usually to identify all of the published and sometimes unpublished literature that relates to your review question so that you can make a careful judgement about what is already known about your topic. In order to do this, your review should be comprehensive and demonstrate a clear method by which you searched for and made sense of the literature you found. This is because you need to be systematic about the approach you take so that you are sure that you have carefully considered all the available literature and have not made vital omissions which might affect the quality of your review. Your research question therefore needs to be clear and to have associated inclusion and exclusion criteria. You need to be able to search for the research and other evidence that is relevant to your review question. You also need to recognize what you find; this might sound like a simple task but it is important that you can distinguish a research paper from a discussion or a paper in which theoretical concepts are discussed, and assess the quality of the papers that seem relevant. You then need to consider an appropriate way of bringing the literature together in an analysis and synthesis. This will lead to your discussion and conclusions, which will either highlight a gap in knowledge that can be a justification for further research or will summarize an existing body of knowledge and hence provide an answer to the question you have set.

You may search for methodological and theoretical literature to support your empirical review. The methodological literature is used to justify your approach to the methods you use in a larger empirical study. The theoretical literature is used to provide a framework for your empirical review or your eventual empirical findings if you are doing a larger study. Hence you need to identify theories that might be relevant to your research topic.

Rather than approaching the literature review as a necessary and possibly somewhat dull component of your study, we want to encourage you to consider the literature review as a crucial and engaging stage of your project which will shape the later stages of your work. To engage fully with the literature at this stage is necessary in order to get to know the background empirical, methodological and theoretical work that has been done in your area. It is not possible to start a project at post-graduate level without being aware of others' work because you need to demonstrate the originality of your research question and explain what your study contributes to the overall body of knowledge on a topic. You need this background analysis of the literature in order to 'pick up the baton' from other researchers, whose work will inform your project in many ways.

In this book we will discuss the different features of the literature review:

- In Chapter 1 we will discuss what a literature review is and why it is important in your post-graduate project.
- In Chapter 2 we will discuss the different types of literature reviews.
- In Chapter 3 we will discuss the inclusion of theoretical, methodological and empirical literature in a literature review and will discuss the role of the research question in shaping the review.
- In Chapter 4 we will discuss how to develop a thorough search strategy which goes beyond simple database searching.
- In Chapter 5 we will discuss how to identify what is relevant to your literature review from the data you have.
- In Chapter 6 we will discuss the role of critical appraisal of the research and other evidence and how critical appraisal can be incorporated into the literature review, according to the approach you are following.
- In Chapter 7 we will discuss how to analyse and synthesize the research and other evidence you have, according to the requirements of the approach to literature review you are following.
- In Chapter 8 we will discuss how to write up your findings and present your literature review.

1

What is a literature review?

In this chapter we will discuss:
- *what a literature review is*
- *the common features of a literature review*
- *why a literature review is important in your post-graduate project*
- *the role a literature review plays in your project*
- *the importance of a focussed question for your review*

What is a literature review?

A literature review is an analysis and synthesis of work that has been undertaken in a particular area: the area that most closely relates to the research question you are exploring for your post-graduate study, be it a small-scale study, master's or a PhD or a doctoral-level award. A literature review involves identifying a question (or questions) which is then answered by the comprehensive and systematic identification, analysis and synthesis of a relevant body of published and sometimes unpublished research and other evidence. The aim of a literature review is to identify what we know and do not know about the question identified. The principles we review in this book apply to all literature reviews; the level of detail to which you apply them will depend on the scope of your individual study.

Literature reviews have become increasingly popular in recent years due to the vast amount of published research and other information associated with the emphasis on evidence-based practice.

A literature review aims to make sense of a body of research and other evidence and presents a summary and analysis of this so that the reader does not have to access and read each individual research report or other material included in the review. This is important because there are increasing amounts of publications and other sources of information available and it is an impossible task to read and assimilate all the information on any one topic. In addition, a well-conducted literature review will provide a critique of the identified research and other evidence and may not include that which is considered to be of poorer quality. This means that when the literature is synthesized together, it is possible to draw conclusions about all the relevant and better-quality research and other evidence. This reduces the likelihood that one misleading research paper will dominate readers' attention and should prevent a 'rogue' piece of evidence from taking centre stage (Harden and Thomas 2005).

Some researchers have commented on the risk that individual pieces of literature, in particular qualitative research studies, are stripped of their context when they are summarized and included in a literature review. These concerns are noted by Thomas and Harden (2008), Noblit and Hare (1988), Pawson et al. (2005) and Sandelowski et al. (1997). However, there is also recognition that without bringing research and other evidence together in a review, individual pieces of research cannot be seen in the context of others. Most researchers agree that bringing the research and other evidence together in a review is a necessary and highly useful task, and the utility of bringing a body of literature together outweighs some of the inevitable 'context stripping'.

There are many different approaches to literature reviewing, which we will discuss throughout this book. Reviews can be composed of all types of published and unpublished research and other material – whatever is relevant to answering the review question.

The common features of a literature review

Although there is a wide range of approaches to literature review, they share many common attributes. If you are undertaking a literature review for a post-graduate award, then the aim of your review will be to present a summary and synthesis of the relevant literature relating to the focus of your specific literature review question(s). While there are many nuances, the overall principles that you will adhere to are largely shown on page 3.

Features that are common to most literature reviews

- Focussed literature review question
- Inclusion and exclusion criteria
- Specific key terms and terms
- List of databases and other sources of evidence
- Record of searches undertaken
- Data extraction in a similar manner from all papers
- Critique and assessment of design and conduct of all literature included
- Presentation of data from all papers
- Analysis and synthesis of the findings in relation to the research question
- Discussion of the extent to which the research question has been answered
- Identification of what is known and what remains unknown
- Standardized method of reporting the review

A clear focus to the review is vital and this is usually achieved by defining a research question (or questions) and related inclusion and exclusion criteria, which determine the remit of the review. Without this, there is a good chance that the focus of the review will 'drift' as interesting but unrelated literature is uncovered. Inclusion and exclusion criteria will enable you to identify research or other evidence that is directly related to answering your review question. Literature that does not meet these criteria can be discarded or be retained in case it provides useful background information.

Searching for relevant research and other evidence is a key aspect in all literature reviews. Reviewers will generally identify key terms which capture the essence of the question they have identified together with a list of potential electronic databases on which to search; however, searching is not limited to a database search. The main focus of the search is likely to be empirical research but you will need to search for other evidence, including methodological and theoretical literature, especially if your literature review is for a doctoral or PhD study. In most cases, the reviewer is searching for all the relevant research that meets the inclusion criteria so that the review is comprehensive and does not make vital omissions. We will discuss this further in Chapter 4.

The search for research and other evidence will inevitably lead you to a wide range of literature and you will need to extract what is relevant for your review, according to the inclusion and exclusion criteria you have identified. Not all of the aspects of all the research or other evidence will be relevant to you and you need to identify what is. There are data extraction (summary) forms that you can develop to assist this process, which we will discuss in Chapter 5.

Once the relevance of the research or other evidence has been established, there are considerations of quality to be made. The literature is likely to be of varying quality and you will need to make a judgement about it and the impact that it will have in your subsequent analysis. This is an area where many methodological differences arise, both in the methods of assessing quality and the decision about the inclusion of research of different qualities in your review. There can be a lack of agreement about what amounts to quality in both the design and conduct of research. For these reasons, it is not always easy to establish the quality of the research or other evidence you have. However, this assessment needs to be made and a judgement is needed as you will generally give more weight to the better designed and conducted research in your subsequent analysis and synthesis. There are also different views on the inclusion of literature of different quality. Some literature reviews include all research that is considered relevant while other reviews exclude research on the basis of their quality (Noyes and Popay 2007; Thomas and Harden 2008). Therefore you may sometimes use lower-quality research if you make the judgement about how and when to include it. If you do not include lower-quality research, you need to justify your decision to exclude it. We will discuss this in Chapter 6. You can determine the strength of evidence most easily if you use an appropriate critical appraisal tool. Appraisal tools are available for virtually all types of evidence that are relevant to your review. We will also discuss this in Chapter 6.

Once you have identified the quality and relevance of the research and other evidence, you need to combine them in an analysis and synthesis of the studies using a suitable method for your review. Data analysis and synthesis are common to all literature reviews, but this is another area where many methodological differences arise. The approach taken will depend on the type of review. If the included research papers are sufficiently similar and use statistics, this can be done numerically, using a statistical calculation often referred to as a meta-analysis. When a meta-analysis is not possible or appropriate, the research or other evidence can be analysed using a non-numerical narrative approach. This is generally a form of thematic analysis and there are many approaches to this, including meta-synthesis, meta-ethnography and thematic analysis. We will discuss this further in Chapter 7.

Finally, there should be an open and transparent reporting of the process of undertaking the review and of the results so that what is known and what remains unknown is clearly communicated and set in the context of your ongoing study. We will discuss this in Chapter 8.

Why is a literature review important for my post-graduate project?

The literature review is important for your post-graduate project because, at this level of study, it is essential that you consider what other academic work exists in the area you are researching and what the strengths and limitations of this work are. It is important that you acknowledge that your work does not exist in isolation and that you can demonstrate how your work relates to the work of others and the contribution of your project to the overall body of knowledge, however modest you consider that to be. You need to come to a conclusion about the contribution made by the existing body of literature to your understanding of your research question. In short, you cannot build your own project without building on the work of others.

However large or small your post-graduate study, you need to consider all the evidence that is relevant to your area of work in a comprehensive and systematic manner. This will be the case whether your entire post-graduate study is literature based or whether you will be reviewing the literature prior to or after undertaking your own empirical study.

Undertaking a structured review is important in order to ensure that you do not overlook a piece of literature which is relevant to your research question in your review. Students are often concerned that they will attend the oral examination or presentation of their work to find that they have omitted a seminal or very significant piece of work from their literature review. This situation is far less likely if you have undertaken a review following a structured approach as we have outlined in the previous section.

Why is there an increasing emphasis on the literature review within my project?

In the last few years, the literature review has been recognized as increasingly important within health and social care generally. We have systematic reviews and summaries of reviews available in clinical practice and on line. This is largely in response to the emphasis on evidence-based practice, the increased amount of research publications and the recognition that, in order to be useful, evidence needs to be assimilated and summarized.

As recognition of the importance of the literature review has increased, so has its role within post-graduate study. In the past, a literature review might have been viewed as something to 'get done' in order to get onto the more interesting task of your own research study. There has been an increased focus on the importance of literature reviews either as a pre-requisite to and therefore shaping an empirical study, or as the main component of the research study itself. Alongside this is the development of a variety of methods that have been designed for doing it. We would encourage all those undertaking a literature review at post-graduate level to consider their method very carefully and to be able to justify the approach they have taken. The process of undertaking a literature review is recognized as a piece of research and the methods of doing so have become as robust as an empirical research study (Whittemore and Knafl 2005; O'Mathuna 2010).

This has not always been the case. If you have accessed master's dissertations and doctoral theses undertaken in previous decades, you are likely to have found a less standardized approach to literature searching and evaluation. You would have generally found a chapter on 'the literature review' but with probably little or no discussion about how the literature search, appraisal and synthesis were undertaken, or why certain papers were selected for review (Dixon-Woods et al. 2007). Research and development in this area have led to an increased understanding of and different approaches to undertaking a literature review together with an acknowledgement that different types of literature reviews are appropriate for different research questions and that rigour can be achieved whichever review method is undertaken.

The influence of the Cochrane Collaboration on the development of the literature review method

One of the most influential factors on the development of research methods for the literature review has been the work of the Cochrane Collaboration. Whether or not the type of literature review you undertake for your project is similar to a 'Cochrane-style' review, this highly systematic approach to the literature review is likely to have influenced the development of method of review that you undertake.

The Cochrane Collaboration was founded in 1992 in Oxford, largely due to the influence of epidemiologist Professor Archie Cochrane (1909–1988). Cochrane was one of the first medical scientists to demonstrate the lack of good evidence upon which many medical treatments and interventions were based. He argued that too much remained unknown about the effectiveness of many treatments and interventions (Cochrane 1972) and proclaimed: 'it is surely a great criticism of our profession [medicine] that we have not organised a critical summary of all relevant randomised controlled trials.' (Cochrane 1979, p. 2).

He challenged the medical community to develop summaries of evidence which would provide guidance for the treatments and interventions given. This challenge resulted in the foundation of the Cochrane Collaboration, which seeks to publish reviews of evidence on the effectiveness of many well-established treatments and interventions. It also gives guidance on the cost effectiveness of treatments and interventions. This work has brought huge developments in the way we manage health care and is ongoing and thriving today. It has also led to the development of the sister organization, the Campbell Collaboration, founded in 2000, which focusses on systematic reviews with a social policy emphasis. The Campbell Collaboration is named after David Campbell, who was a member of the National Academy of Science in the United States and who advocated that social policy should be based on sound scientific experiment.

One early systematic review demonstrated how the standardized review process can provide potentially life-saving information. Mulrow (1994) describes a systematic review of 33 studies which looked at the effectiveness of streptokinase in the treatment of acute myocardial infarction (heart attack). Streptokinase, although now well known as a life-saving drug, was at that time not routinely administered to patients following a myocardial infarction due to lack of evidence about its effectiveness. There were many small randomized controlled trials (RCTs) which compared the outcomes of patients who were given streptokinase and those who were not, but the results were inconclusive due to the size of the studies. However when the results of these studies were pooled in a meta-analysis (a statistical procedure which combines the results of all similar studies), the true effect of the streptokinase became apparent, which had not been identifiable prior to the meta-analysis. This review revolutionalized care of patients following myocardial infarction, and Mulrow comments that this benefit could have been demonstrated 20 years previously (and saved many lives) if the meta-analysis had been undertaken much earlier.

Another systematic review which revolutionized practice was undertaken by Gilbert et al. (2005) who undertook a systematic review that identified equally life-saving information. This team of researchers reviewed the evidence about widely held beliefs that babies should sleep on their stomachs. This public health advice, which had been published in many popular child health textbooks, dated back to the 1960s. In reviewing available research, the researchers found evidence that this advice was incorrect. Gilbert et al. estimate that as many as 10 000 babies' lives could have been saved if an earlier systematic review of this evidence had been undertaken.

As you can see from the examples above, the Cochrane Collaboration systematic reviews are concerned with determining the effectiveness of treatments and care procedures. It is widely agreed that if you are concerned with the effectiveness of an intervention, then the best way to find out about this is to undertake an RCT. For this reason most Cochrane Collaboration systematic reviews incorporate RCTs. Other literature reviews which have a different focus will incorporate a variety of research designs.

What is an RCT?
This is an approach to an experiment in which one intervention is compared against another or no intervention. Participants who have agreed to enter an experiment are allocated at random into one of two or more groups. The different groups will receive a different treatment or intervention. At the end of the experiment, the effect of each intervention or treatment will be measured on the participants in each group and the differences in outcomes between the participants in different groups will be compared. The

principle is that, due to the random assignment of the treatment, all other influencing factors have been equalled out and any difference between the participants in the different groups can be put down to the different treatment or interventions. RCTs have less systematic bias about the effects of an intervention or treatment and data can be analysed statistically. For this reason, RCTs are generally used to answer research questions about the effect of an intervention or treatment (for example, the effect of a drug or sleeping position). Although there is general agreement that this type of experiment is the best way to determine whether or not a treatment or intervention is effective, in any health or social care discipline, some researchers argue that there should be an element of caution about this approach. For example, Pawson et al. (2005), Greenhalgh (2014) and Borgerson (2009) argue that simple experiments should not be used to evaluate complex interventions and, when they are, this can lead to the over-simplification of results.

Systematic approach to a wider range of literature review questions

Cochrane Collaboration systematic reviews follow a very detailed method, which we will refer to throughout this book. The interest in and development of the Cochrane Collaboration systematic review was accompanied by interest in a more systematic approach to literature reviews more generally. This has led to an expansion of ideas and approaches to comprehensive and systematic reviews of the literature, which may differ in method from the original Cochrane Collaboration approach but whose aims and intentions will be similar (Grant and Booth 2009).

The discussion and focus on the importance of the literature review have re-energized the process of doing a literature review, particularly at post-graduate level, and we will discuss a number of different methods throughout this book. What is important is that the researcher develops a systematic and comprehensive approach to the search, appraisal, analysis and synthesis of the research and other material, within the scope that his or her study allows. This should include reference to rigour, transparency and replicability of the method of undertaking the literature review.

Clarification of terminology

You can see from the stages discussed on page 3 that most literature reviews follow a systematic and comprehensive approach. Possibly the most comprehensive approach is the systematic review, which is a specific method of undertaking a literature review which we discuss later in this chapter. Clarity about the use of terms is important. All literature reviews should follow a systematic approach and you are encouraged to adopt a systematic approach to any type of literature review you embark on. In other words, your review will be systematic even if it does not adhere to the detail of what is formally referred to as a systematic review and may in fact be more closely aligned with another method of review. The point to remember is that your review should be done systematically whether or not you are specifically undertaking a systematic review.

You might find also find that the term 'meta-analysis' – a term used to refer to the statistical analysis of the results from individual research studies within a systematic review – is used to describe a systematic review that includes a meta-analysis (Saba et al. 2014).

What role will a literature review play in my project?

There are many different roles that the literature review might play and many different types of literature review that you might use. This will depend on your individual research project and you will establish the role of your literature review in your study during discussion with your supervisor or supervisory team. For most research projects at post-graduate level, the literature review will fall into one of these two categories (Table 1.1):

- supportive literature review
- standalone literature review

Supportive literature review

This is the classic approach to the literature review. It is undertaken prior to an empirical study, often as part of a PhD or master's or a much larger funded study. The purpose of the literature review is to inform the

Table 1.1 The role of the literature review in your research project

	The research question is **answered** by a comprehensive and systematic literature review.	The research project is **supported** by a comprehensive and systematic literature review.
Your main project is an empirical study. The literature review will consider what we already know about the topic and justify your research question. We will refer to this as a **supportive literature review.**		✔
Your main project is a literature review from which you hope to answer a research question. We will refer to this as a **standalone literature review.**	✔	

researchers of all relevant previous work that has been done in an area. This will often focus on what other empirical research has been undertaken in the area but will also draw on other types of literature, such as theoretical and methodological literature. It helps to identify what is known and what is unknown about the topic of your research. There is a caveat here, however, as in certain approaches to qualitative research, for example grounded theory, the literature review may be undertaken after the main study has been completed so as not to influence or lead the initial analysis.

Standalone literature review

This is a more recent type of literature review in which the intention of the review is to answer a research question rather than to identify a gap in knowledge that leads to further research, although these reviews often do point to the need for further research. The methods for undertaking this approach have been the focus of much scrutiny in recent years due to the attention given to this method by the Cochrane Collaboration and the development of the systematic review. While not all literature reviews which attempt to address a research question as their main purpose use a Cochrane-style systematic review method, most strive for a systematic approach. This type of review is helpful when you need to evaluate the contribution of the existing literature to knowledge in a particular area: for example, on the most appropriate interventions or services to commission.

The importance of a focussed literature review question

Whichever role the literature review plays in your research, it is important that your research is led by a focussed question. If you have several different sections of your literature review, each is likely to be led by a different question, which will have a specific focus.

Therefore, it is important to identify a focussed literature review question so that the aims and scope of your review are clear from the outset. This might sound very obvious, but one of the common pitfalls for those undertaking a literature review is a lack of clarity about the aims and purpose of the review. This is important as otherwise you will risk going 'off track' and including literature which is interesting but irrelevant to the aims of your review. Many students commence their literature review lacking clarity about what they need to achieve and hence fail to include the most appropriate research or other evidence and subsequently waste a lot of time and effort. Without a clear question, there is also the risk that you will drift from the main aims of the review while the review is in progress. As a result the review might be vague and not meet the needs of the project.

Associated with the development of a clear question is the development of clear inclusion and exclusion criteria which provide a detailed guide to the literature that will be relevant to your review. Inclusion and exclusion criteria allow you as the researcher to be very specific about the type of literature you will include. We will discuss this further when we discuss searching for literature in Chapter 4.

Sometimes the literature review question will be a simple deductive question. This assumes that the 'answer' can be found in research or other evidence by a simple deductive process. The terms used to describe the literature review question are likely to be unambiguous and clearly defined in the existing work available. For example, a literature review question might seek to find out about evidence of the effectiveness of topical antibiotics in treating impetigo in young children. For most literature review questions, it is important that you can define the terms used in the literature review question. In this case, the terms 'effectiveness' and 'young children' would need to be clearly defined so that the researcher has clarity about the focus of the review and that this clarity is then present in the review.

At times, however, the purpose of the literature review may be to clarify and develop concepts (Dixon-Woods et al. 2005). For these types of reviews, it may not be possible to clearly define the terms used, which might initially be 'tentative, fuzzier and contested' (Greenhalgh et al. 2005, p. 418). A concept analysis is an example of an approach to reviewing published material in order to clarify the working use of a term. For example, a literature review question might seek to consider how a concept is discussed in published material. Autonomy is an example of a concept that might mean different things to different people and so is not easy to define, and it was the subject of a concept analysis undertaken by Lindberg et al. (2014).

The role that your literature review plays in your project might have an influence on the literature review question. If your main project is a standalone literature review and you intend to answer a specific question through an analysis of the research and other relevant evidence, then the focus of your literature review question is likely to be the same as the focus of your entire project. While you are also likely to refer to the methodological literature to justify the approach you took in the design of your review and the theoretical literature in order to develop the theories that relate to your review, the main focus of your review will be the literature that directly answers your literature review question.

If your main project is an empirical study, your study is likely to be supported by one or more literature reviews: for example, an empirical literature review of what is already known about the focus of your study, in addition to a review of theoretical and empirical literature relating to different aspects of the research question and how it is going to be answered. Each of these sections is likely to have a different question.

The important point is that your literature review must be focussed around a specific question which is relevant for your project. Your question will be supported by inclusion and exclusion criteria which will guide your search for relevant research and other information, which we will discuss in Chapter 4.

In summary

In this chapter we have described what a literature review is and the common features that are present in most reviews. We have also described the role that a literature review might play in your post-graduate study. At the start of your review, you need to identify whether your literature review will be a standalone review or a pre-requisite to a larger empirical study and this may have a subtle effect on the way you approach your review, as portrayed in Table 1.1. It is vital to have a clearly focussed question for your literature review otherwise the review is likely to become unfocussed. The research question and associated inclusion and exclusion criteria will direct the focus of the review.

We have argued that the importance of the literature review in your post-graduate project has increased in recent years and that this is related to the increased importance and significance of the role of the literature review within the health and social care more generally. While it has always been important to set your work within the context of others', the methods of doing so have recently become more diverse, explicit and rigorous. In the next chapter we will discuss the different approaches to undertaking a literature review.

Key points

- A literature review is an analysis and synthesis of work undertaken in an area.
- It is important to set your work within the context of others'.
- The methods for undertaking a literature review have developed in recent years.
- There are features that are common to most literature reviews.
- Your review might be a standalone review or supportive to a larger study.
- It is important to have a clearly focussed question for your review.

2

Different methods for doing a literature review

In this chapter we will discuss:
- *Different methods of doing a literature review*
- *Examples of projects where different methods have been used*

Once you have established the role that the literature review will play in your study and the focus of your literature review question, you need to consider the most appropriate method for your review. There are many different types of literature review methods. Some are concerned with the synthesis of quantitative research, others with examining qualitative research and others with a combination of the two. Some use qualitative methods of analysis and synthesis and others use quantitative statistical methods.

There is no ideal type of literature review method (Arksey and O'Malley 2005) and all can be conducted with a rigorous method; you should choose the one that best fits the literature and their study and you must be ready to defend your choice in your written dissertation or viva.

Some methods of undertaking a literature review are clearly more complex than others and some are more suited to different areas of study than others. There are also some which can be undertaken by novice researchers and others which are recommended for those with more expertise (Thorne et al. 2004; Finlayson and Dixon 2008). For example, some of the approaches to reviewing the literature require a team of researchers to complete, such as using a detailed systematic review method like that undertaken by the Cochrane Collaboration. However, there are ways that you can adapt these approaches and we will explore how potentially complex methods can be adapted and used appropriately and realistically at post-graduate-level study.

Different approaches to your literature review

In this section we will discuss a range of approaches you might consider using, depending on the needs of your study and the role that the literature review plays in your research. Any of these approaches can be used whether your literature review is a standalone study or a pre-requisite to a larger review, although the time and word limit you have for your review will influence the approach you take and the detail with which you are able to carry out the review. You may follow one of the methods we describe in this chapter or you may follow the general principles of a literature review without adhering to a specific method. If you decide to focus on one of the approaches in a larger-scale review, we advise that you access the additional references we have given which fully describe the method. Some of the approaches can be used for the review of empirical research only while others combine the review of empirical, theoretical and other literature.

Table 2.1 Different types of literature reviews

Systematic review with meta-analysis
Incorporating quantitative research, often supplemented by a quantitative narrative synthesis

Systematic review with meta-aggregation
Incorporating qualitative research where results are pooled together

Systematic review with an interpretation: meta-ethnography, thematic synthesis, meta-synthesis
Incorporating qualitative research where results are re-interpreted

Systematic review of mixed methods studies with interpretation: critical interpretative synthesis, integrative reviews
Incorporating mixed methods research where results are re-interpreted

Systematic reviews to develop theory: realist reviews, narrative synthesis
Incorporating mixed methods research to develop theory

Systematically undertaken overviews: scoping studies, bibliometric analysis
Incorporating all studies but focussing on searching rather than appraisal or analysis

Systematic review with a meta-analysis

We will start with the original systematic review method. We call this the 'original systematic review' because the first systematic reviews were designed to include a meta-analysis, or statistical analysis, of the results of all the included studies in order to determine the effectiveness of a treatment or intervention as discussed earlier. Since then, systematic reviews have developed to include a variety of methods of analysis, but systematic review with a meta-analysis was the original design of this type of review.

The method for undertaking a systematic review with meta-analysis is described and available online in the Cochrane Collaboration *Handbook*, which was first published in 1994. In this and subsequent editions, the exacting methods of undertaking a Cochrane-style systematic review have been developed and established, and they are well documented in the latest edition of the handbook (Higgins and Green 2011).

A systematic review with a meta-analysis is a very structured and detailed process. It is usually undertaken by a review team so that more than one person performs each task to enhance the accuracy and reliability of the process. The researchers may be assisted by an advisory group, which can include patient and client representatives.

A systematic review aims to identify, evaluate and undertake a statistical re-analysis of data from all the existing studies that refer to a specific research question and that meet specific inclusion and exclusion criteria. For those undertaking a Cochrane Collaboration systematic review, the literature review question is usually focussed on a question about the effectiveness of an intervention. Other systematic reviews or meta-analysis may have a focus other than that of effectiveness.

One main feature of a systematic review is the effort which is expended in identifying relevant studies for inclusion. The search goes far beyond electronic subject-specific database searches and extends to the location of unpublished papers and other evidence, which we discuss in detail in Chapter 4. The focus of the review is tightly controlled; studies that are interesting but not relevant are often excluded from the review. Studies are assessed for bias; most systematic review protocols have criteria for assessment of bias which means that those studies that are relevant but of high risk of bias are excluded from the review. It is possible for researchers to identify many studies which are relevant only to reject these studies a little further down the line due to concern about the quality of their design and/or conduct. It is therefore not uncommon for researchers to conclude that there is insufficient evidence to answer the research question they set out to address in their systematic review.

The design of the review is written up in advance of performing it, in a protocol which might be published or registered with a register of systematic reviews such as PROSPERO. Protocols ensure transparency, and if more than one person is involved with the review it helps to ensure that everyone is following the same steps. There are many excellent texts which report in detail the process of undertaking a systematic review (Centre for Reviews and Dissemination 2008; Higgins and Green 2011; Bettany-Saltikov 2012; Chandler and Hopewell 2013).

Understanding the impact of systematic reviews

The systematic review and meta-analysis are generally viewed to be a great scientific advancement of our time. They have enabled scientists and the medical community to state with certainty what works and what does not, or what is effective and what is not, in terms of treatments and screening interventions, thus helping decision-making for screening and treatment options. However, the process is not necessarily straightforward. In 2011, the Nordic Cochrane group published a systematic review in which their analysis showed that mammograms were not effective in reducing the mortality rate from breast cancer (Gøtzsche and Nielsen 2011). These findings provoked intense discussion among scientists and the medical community, and when the papers were re-analysed, omitting some of the older papers from the meta-analysis (Marmot et al. 2012), the results were more encouraging. Hence it remains a judgement call as to which studies are included in the analysis and the consequences of this.

Even if we accept the need for informed judgement, more fundamentally, the systematic review and the RCT, which is often selected within a systematic review, are not without their critics. For example, Seers (2007) expresses concern that data might not be as context free as we might like to think and that results from RCTs might imply a robustness of the results that may not exist in reality. Pawson et al. (2005) suggest that RCTs should be considered with caution for all but very simple interventions and should have limited use in contemporary studies of complex interventions. They argue that RCTs are often not appropriate in a social setting where it is not possible to do a 'clean policy on/policy off comparison' (p. 51).

As a result, Pawson et al. (2005) argue that the results of many Cochrane-style reviews which include a meta-analysis can be over-simplified and that the rigorous process of a systematic review, which excludes certain studies, eliminates contextual details, selectively utilizes findings and takes averages of effects so that eventually 'so much is winnowed away that the meta-analysis is left with only a few studies that pass methodological muster' (pp. 42–3). Pawson et al. (2005) are also particularly critical of systematic reviews which attempt to combine data in a meta-analysis from disparate studies. They argue that unless studies are conducted in exceptionally similar settings, with similar context and participants, the results cannot be meaningfully pooled in a meta-analysis. They relate this in particular to social programmes (although the same can be said for medical programmes and interventions) – that whether the complex intervention works is dependent on who seeks them out, who delivers them, whether they tell others about them and a variety of other factors. Hence any attempt to pool the data from studies which look at similar but not identical interventions is likely to be flawed and stripped of meaning. However, the Cochrane Collaboration do not recommend that results are just a pooled estimate of effect. Instead they require a narrative critique of the included papers together with an acknowledgement of the limitations of pooling results such as the level of heterogeneity (or differences) between participants or interventions.

Examples of systematic reviews with meta-analysis

Examples of systematic reviews can be found at www.cochrane.org and www.campbellcollaboration.org. If there are many systematic reviews and the topic seems to be well studied, you may come across a review of reviews. For example Greaves et al. (2011) undertook a review of the published systematic reviews which looked at the effectiveness of dietary and lifestyle interventions changes for adults at risk of type 2 diabetes.

When might a systematic review with meta-analysis be appropriate for your post-graduate study?

A systematic review with meta-analysis may be appropriate if you are reviewing studies using quantitative designs which fulfil the criteria to combine in a meta-analysis. Systematic reviews with a meta-analysis have been undertaken at PhD or doctoral-level study and sometimes at master's level work, and the process can be adapted to suit your level of experience and resources. For example, the role of the team of researchers and advisory group usually associated with a systematic review project can be carried out by members of your supervisory team, and peers or colleagues who may be prepared to become involved with your work and assist you in making decisions about the conduct of your systematic review, thus enhancing its rigour. It is therefore advisable to find at least one academic within your discipline who is willing to duplicate some of the tasks you need to carry out when undertaking the review as this will increase the accuracy of your review and make it more publishable. We will discuss the tasks where this is possible throughout this book.

For example, Taylor et al. (2014) undertook a systematic review and meta-analysis to examine the mental health of people who had quitted smoking and compared their mental health with those who continued to smoke. In an email correspondence, Taylor explained why they had used a systematic review with meta-analysis:

> *When we reviewed the theories and concepts around what happens to people's mental health when they quit smoking, we found opposing explanations. We chose a systematic review with meta-analysis to allow us to look at the empirical research that had been carried out in order to quantify the changes in mental health in those who stopped smoking and those who continued to smoke. This enabled us to see which explanations were supported by empirical research. A benefit of this approach was that it allowed us to determine if the average 'effect' was different between different study designs (for example randomised or observational) different methods used in the studies (for example, short versus long follow-up), or different populations (for example people with depression compared with people from the general population).*
>
> *My supervisors adopted a very hands-on approach and helped with most tasks, including checking papers for inclusion/exclusion, data extraction, analysis and interpretation. Generally speaking at each major stage of the study we had a supervisory meeting to discuss progress and the next steps forward, and sought further advice from our peers when appropriate*
>
> (Taylor 2015, via email)

Systematic review with a narrative synthesis

In addition to a meta-analysis, a quantitative narrative synthesis – to be distinguished from the mixed-method approach to narrative synthesis discussed later in this chapter – can be used. Pope et al. (2007) describe a quantitative narrative synthesis as the description, explanation and interpretation of the study findings and the attempt to find explanations for the findings, which enhance the interpretation of the meta-analysis. In a quantitative narrative synthesis, the results of the systematic review are described and discussed textually, with a focus on the context and study characteristics in order to develop a richer, in-depth understanding of the results than that presented in the statistics provided by the meta-analysis. Narrative synthesis is often undertaken alongside a traditional systematic review, for example Rock et al. (2015) and Sampson et al. (2014).

Alternative types of systematic review

The term systematic review is not reserved exclusively for reviews produced by the Cochrane or Campbell Collaboration, and systematic reviews are often undertaken to address literature review questions that do not address questions of effectiveness. When in this situation, the research papers in the review cannot be summarized in a meta-analysis, and a different approach to analysis and synthesis is used.

When a systematic review with a meta-analysis is not appropriate for your study – for example, you may have data which are insufficient for the calculation of effect sizes, or you have qualitative studies or a wide range of qualitative and quantitative research – there are many other approaches to literature review which you can consider. Your decision will depend on the types of papers which you have and the level of analysis you intend to undertake.

Most of these approaches contain the common features of a literature review as presented on page 3 in Chapter 1; however, there are many subtle differences which you will take into account if you follow one of these methods. The different methods of literature review vary according to the methods of searching, critical appraisal, and analysis. Some reviews aim to pool and combine the results of the literature and summarize what the different studies are saying while others aim for interpretation. It can be argued that qualitative research is complex to combine in a review as there are different philosophical underpinnings to the different qualitative methods used and there is the risk of a loss of context if these approaches are combined. However, the risk of this is generally not considered to outweigh the benefit of undertaking a review but should be considered when any review is undertaken.

Systematic review with a meta-aggregation or pooling of results

Meta-aggregative approaches

The meta-aggregative review was developed by researchers at the Joanna Briggs Institute in Australia as a response to the need to develop a method for the analysis and synthesis of qualitative research which cannot be analysed within a meta-analysis. In the Reviewers' Manual for the Joanna Briggs Institute (2014), meta-aggregation is described as a method that mirrors the process of a quantitative review, while holding onto the traditions and requirements of qualitative research.

In a meta-aggregative review, papers are searched for according to clear inclusion and exclusion criteria and critically appraised. Data analysis and synthesis involves the aggregation of evidence using themes rather than statistics, and the aim of the review is a summary of the themes identified in the papers included in the review. Meta-aggregative reviews are described as the assembly and combination of many research findings into a whole that is more than the sum of the individual parts.

The meta-aggregative approach is described as one that emphasizes the complexities of the research while providing a synthesis that is transparent and that results in synthesized statements which are practical and usable (Hannes and Lockwood 2011), an attribute which, it is argued, makes this approach attractive to policy makers and practitioners. Indeed, Hannes and Lockwood (2011) refer to meta-aggregation as a pragmatic approach, citing the work of John Dewey (1938) and his understanding of pragmatism as 'the meaning of any thought or idea are determined by the practical usefulness' (p. 1636).

> **Examples of a systematic review with meta-aggregation** are available on the Joanna Briggs Institute website: www.joannabriggs.edu.au/pubs/systematic_reviews.php.

When might a meta-aggregative review be appropriate for your post-graduate study?

For those considering a meta-aggregative approach to their literature review, Hannes and Lockwood (2011) argue that concepts need to be well developed rather than exploratory and in the analysis researchers should be aiming for a clear and transparent relationship between the participants' experience and the related themes (p. 1636). This is because the aim of meta-aggregation is to summarize rather than to interpret, and to achieve a pragmatic and reliable representation of the themes arising in the literature.

For example, Jakimowicz et al. (2015) undertook an aggregative literature review to investigate the factors that impact upon patients' subjective experiences of nurse-led clinics. In their study, they provide a rationale for why they chose an aggregative approach:

> *This study aimed to systematically review the qualitative evidence on factors that affect the experience of patients attending nurse-led clinics and compare with key elements of person-centred care. Limiting the study to qualitative literature allowed the capture of experiential research focused on the essence of the 'experience' of the patient. The Joanna Briggs Institute (JBI) methodology of meta-aggregation was used. This method provides a high quality synthesis of primary qualitative research and delivers evidence of what is currently known, recommendations for practice and future research as well as what remains unknown on the topic. The method evolved from the work of Estabrooks et al. (1994) and Sandelowski et al. (1997) and unlike other methods of qualitative synthesis does not aim to reinterpret data.*
>
> (Jakimowicz et al. 2015, p. 20)

The meta-aggregative approach can be regarded as the qualitative equivalent to a meta-analysis. The results of the studies are pooled together so that the findings of ten studies are stronger than the findings of one study.

 # Systematic review of qualitative studies with an interpretative focus

For those undertaking a literature review in which their aim is not to summarize but to interpret, there are methods which facilitate the further interpretation of the data. Some methods are specific to the analysis of qualitative methods and some can be used with mixed methods.

Meta-ethnography was developed by Noblit and Hare (1988) as an alternative to the pragmatic summary and aggregation of themes identified in a review. Meta-ethnography was one of the first documented approaches to the analysis of qualitative research and represents a move away from meta-aggregation. The aim of a meta-ethnography is not the combination of the results of qualitative data but the search for new interpretations from the data. The features involved in a meta-ethnography are similar to those described on page 3, but in the analysis there is a focus on interpretation, rather than on providing a simple summary of the data. For those undertaking an interpretative analysis, the results are:

> *integrations that are more than the sum of the parts, in that they offer novel interpretations of findings. These interpretations will not be found in any one research report but rather are inferences derived from taking all of the reports in a sample as a whole.*
>
> Sandelowski (2004, p. 1358)

Despite the name given to this method and the initial focus on the interpretation of ethnographic studies, the authors advised that their approach was not limited to the analysis and synthesis of ethnographic studies and could be used far more extensively to analyse a wide range of qualitative research studies. However a meta-ethnography does not include quantitative studies.

In order to emphasize the inclusivity of this interpretative approach, further adaptations of meta-ethnography were developed: **meta-interpretation** (Finfgeld 1999), **thematic synthesis** (Thomas and Harden 2008) and **meta-synthesis** (Stern and Harris 1985; Walsh and Downe 2005). These approaches share the common features of a literature review as described on page 3 but they emphasize that all qualitative studies can be included, rather than just ethnographic studies. These approaches are based on the original work of Noblit and Hare (1988).

An example of a systematic review with an interpretative approach

The Cochrane Collaboration recently published its first qualitative systematic review (Glenton et al. 2013), which used an interpretative approach to examine the barriers to and facilitators of the implementation of lay health workers to improve access to maternal and child health services.

When might an interpretative approach for the review of qualitative studies be appropriate for your post-graduate study?

Although Noblit and Hare (1988) argue that the meta-ethnographic approach is not for the novice, this interpretative approach might be appropriate when you aim to explore and interpret concepts in detail rather than simply report and summarize the findings of a range of studies. They are useful when the concepts explored in a review are difficult to define and require further clarification within the review. An interpretative approach can only be used with qualitative studies.

For example, Satink et al. (2013) undertook an interpretative approach, using a thematic synthesis to explore patients' views on the impact of stroke. In email correspondence, Satink explained the rationale for this:

> *We used a thematic synthesis as we wanted to focus on the client's perspective of the impact of stroke on their role and their view of 'self', and we only wanted to include qualitative studies. A mixed method could have been included if it was possible to extract specifically data about the clients' perspective. We chose an interpretative approach as we wanted to go further than just a summary of the data. Whilst a summary is interesting, we wanted to undertake additional analysis and interpretation, based on the different findings from the different primary qualitative studies. This involved looking at the 60–70 themes that were described in the primary qualitative studies. We then undertook an additional analysis in order to develop new 'overarching' themes. To strengthen the evidence for the new overarching themes, quotations from the primary studies have been used in the description of the findings. Moreover, we have put in a chart which shows which primary studies we have used for the new overarching themes. With this synthesis of qualitative research, we have given a stronger voice to patients' perspectives than individual studies do.*

(Satink 2015, via email)

 # Systematic review of qualitative and quantitative studies with an interpretative focus

Despite initial concern about combining qualitative and quantitative research in a literature review due to different methodological considerations (Jensen and Allen 1996; Rogers et al. 1996), there has been increasing recognition that research from a diverse range of research methods may be relevant to a particular research question and should therefore be examined within one literature review.

Harden and Thomas (2005) argue that research questions should not be confined in their answers by the type of study but by relevance of the study to the research question and hence incorporate a range of study designs in their reviews. Thus recent developments have seen approaches that advocate the combination of different types of research and other evidence, including theoretical evidence.

The integrative review is an approach that incorporates the integration of a wide range of literature in a review rather than just qualitative methods and was developed by Whittemore and Knafl (2005). The integrative review is described as the broadest type of review that allows for the inclusion of experimental and non-experimental research in addition to theoretical literature. A diverse range of literature can therefore be included in an integrative review. The integrative review outlines the features of a literature review as presented on page 3. A comprehensive search is followed by data extraction and critical appraisal. The aim of the analysis is the thorough and unbiased interpretation of primary sources, along with an innovative synthesis (Whittemore and Knalf 2005). The integrative review can be used to define concepts, review theories and analyse methods (Whittemore and Knafl 2005) in addition to the analysis of empirical research to address clinically relevant question (Flemming 2010; Niela-Vilén et al. 2014).

Critical interpretative synthesis is another approach that incorporates a wide range of literature in an interpretative review. Critical interpretative synthesis was developed by Dixon-Woods et al. (2006) and is closely based on meta-ethnography and the work of Noblit and Hare (1988) with reference to grounded theory. The aim of critical interpretative synthesis is the generation of a theory and the developments of new concepts, so it is a more focussed approach than the integrative review. For this reason, the methods involved in critical interpretative synthesis reflect those used in a grounded theory, for example the inductive forming of the review question and theoretical sampling for included literature. Dixon-Woods et al. (2006) describe how, in their qualitative review of the literature, they initially set out to use a meta-ethnographic approach but found that this approach did not seem suitable for their study of a large number of disparate studies, including quantitative studies. As a result, the researchers adapted the meta-ethnography technique to one that incorporated the use of a wide range of studies but which retained the essence of constant comparative analysis and interpretation. This also facilitated the development of theory. Dixon-Woods et al. (2006) argue that since the generation of theory is often based on a broad range of evidence, not just empirical research studies, non-research evidence should be included in the synthesis if appropriate.

Examples of a mixed-method review

Niela-Vilén et al. (2014) used an integrative approach to a literature review to investigate Internet peer support for new parents.

Flemming (2010) used a critical interpretative synthesis when reviewing a diverse range of research literature in her review to explore use of morphine to treat cancer pain.

When might an interpretative approach to the review of a mixed method of qualitative and quantitative studies be appropriate for your post-graduate study?

A mixed-method approach to your literature review might be appropriate when you have a combination of research designs that are relevant to your research question rather than literature which fits into either a 'quantitative' or 'qualitative' design category.

For example, Niela-Vilén et al. (2014) undertook an integrative review to investigate the use of an Internet peer support for new parents. In an email correspondence, Niela-Vilén explained the rational for using an integrative approach to the review:

> *I think the reason for selecting the integrative review was quite practical. Based on the preliminary literature search it was clear that the relevant studies had different methodologies so we needed an approach that could incorporate different types of studies, although we restricted this to research studies only (rather than non research papers). We based our review on the methodological paper by Whittemore & Knafl (2005) which is quite easy to follow and provides an understandable framework.*

(Niela-Vilén 2015, via email)

 ## Systematic approaches to literature review which emphasize the role of theory

---

Narrative synthesis of mixed methods – not to be confused with a narrative synthesis of quantitative data as described earlier – is an approach that emphasizes the role of theory within the review, but its aim is primarily to develop an understanding of the empirical studies rather than the development of theory. Those undertaking a narrative synthesis commence their review with the identification of relevant theories that underpin the question they are reviewing. After defining a research review question, the reviewers follow the features of a literature review identified earlier: searching for literature, extracting relevant information, appraising the quality of the information, followed by an analysis and synthesis. The narrative synthesis approach described by Popay et al. (2006) offers a wide variety of approaches to analysis and synthesis of literature including descriptions, tabulating data, content analysis, thematic analysis, concept and ideas mapping, and qualitative case descriptions.

When might a narrative synthesis be appropriate for your post-graduate study?

A narrative synthesis might be appropriate for your review when you have a combination of research designs and where you are interested in exploring these in relation to established theories and concepts.

For example, Dunleavy is currently undertaking a narrative synthesis review to explore the barriers to and facilitators of the recruitment of patients and carers into randomized controlled trials in palliative care. In an email correspondence, Dunleavy explained the rational for using a narrative synthesis approach to the review:

> An initial scope of the literature showed that there is limited primary research addressing my research question. However, researchers have written about their experiences of recruitment either in specific articles looking at this issue or in the discussion sections of primary palliative care randomized controlled trial papers. My review is based on the premise that narrative observations will provide a valuable insight into what the barriers and facilitators are to patient and carer recruitment to palliative care randomised controlled clinical trials. I have chosen the narrative synthesis approach outlined by Popay et al. 2006, as it 'adopts a textual approach to the process of synthesis' (Popay et al. 2006 p 5), it will allow me to include a wider variety of 'evidence' including narrative observations as well as primary research to answer my review question and it provides a general framework to guide the synthesis process which can include the use of theory.

> (Dunleavy 2015, via email)

The meta-narrative method is another approach that incorporates the integration of a wide range of literature but which emphasizes the importance of the theoretical background of the studies within the review. The meta-narrative approach was developed by Greenhalgh et al. (2005) and Pope and Mays (2006). Meta-narrative reviews draw on the work of Kuhn (1962), who argues that scientific paradigms evolve over time and research should be considered within the paradigm within which it was conducted. A meta-narrative review explores the paradigm in addition to the research which has been identified as relevant to the review. In order to incorporate research from different research traditions, in a meta-narrative approach, research is compared initially from within its own paradigm so that any inconsistencies within the data could be explored within the paradigm in which it was generated.

The realist review is an approach to the literature review which is primarily concerned with the development of theory. The realist review was first developed by Pawson et al. (2005) as an approach to developing understanding about why complex interventions might work rather than accepting the findings of the systematic review with meta-analysis at face value. The realist review is concerned with identifying causes for why complex interventions might work on the principle that 'what causes something to happen has nothing to do with the number of times we observe it happening' (Sayer 2000, p. 14).

The purpose of a realist review is to explore why a programme or intervention works rather than just to ask the question 'does it work?' The aim is explanation and in particular an exploration of the theories that underlie an intervention. The purpose is to articulate the underlying theories, 'what works for whom and in what circumstances' (Pawson et al. 2005, p. 74). The realist review has the same common features of a literature review but has the search for underlying theories as a central component of its search strategy. The aim of the review is the generation of theory. The approach is currently developmental although it has been widely used in health and social care (Wong et al. 2013a, 2013b).

Examples of a realist review

An example of a realist review is McCormack et al. (2013), which examined the role of change agents in the implementation of an evidence-based practice approach. In this review, researchers were interested in the role change agents play in the promotion of evidence-based practice and why this was important. The review identified that accessibility of the change agent, its cultural compatibility and attitude all contributed to the promotion of evidence-based practice in addition to an emphasis on reflection on practice.

When might a realist review be appropriate for your post-graduate study?

A realist review is a complex review and might be used when your study is a standalone literature review. The methods for undertaking a realist review are still developing and you would need to explore these as you undertake yours.

Atherton et al. undertook a conceptual review drawing on realist methods to identify explanations of why and how various alternatives to the face-to-face consultations with healthcare professionals might or might not work. The researchers were interested in drawing on consultations between different population groups in different settings. In an email correspondence, Atherton explained the choice of realist methods for this review:

> *We chose to use realist methods in completing our review because it allowed us to answer important questions on 'how' and 'why' these alternatives might work – questions that are not possible to address using a systematic review with a meta-analysis. The method provided a framework for identifying and managing the syntheses of research of different types. We based our review on the conceptual review by Ziebland and Wyke 2012 (www.ncbi.nlm.nih.gov/pmc/articles/ PMC3460203), which clearly outlines the approach to this type of work*
> (Atherton 2015, via email)

 # Overview literature review

Some literature reviews are designed to provide an overview of literature in an area and are often a pre-requisite of a more specific literature review.

Scoping study review

A scoping study review is an approach that incorporates the use of all types of research and other evidence in a review (Arksey and O'Malley

2005). This is a versatile and flexible approach to a review, the aim of which is to map key areas of research or the use of concepts: for example, how particular terms are used and for what purposes (Mays et al. 2005). Scoping studies can be the precursor to a detailed literature review and are generally less detailed than the other literature review methods referred to in this chapter. A scoping study will usually involve the identification of a research question and broad searching strategy, followed by the charting and summarizing of the data. Literature is not generally omitted from the review according to quality criteria and there is no attempt to weight the evidence. According to Arksey and O'Malley (2005), 'this is because the scoping study does not seek to assess the quality of evidence and consequently cannot determine whether particular studies provide robust and generalizable findings' (Arksey and O'Malley 2005, p. 27).

Literature is summarized rather than synthesized. Arksey and O'Malley argue:

> *the scoping study does not address the issue of synthesis, that is the relative weight of evidence in favour of the effectiveness of any particular intervention . . . consequently scoping studies provide a narrative or descriptive account of available research*

(Arksey and O'Mally 2005, p. 30)

Example of a scoping study
An example of a scoping study is Arksey and O'Malley (2005), who reviewed the literature on the effectiveness and cost effectiveness of services to support people with mental health problems. The authors' aim was to achieve a comprehensive (rather than detailed) coverage of the main findings. Results were collated and summarized to present an overview of all the material reviewed.

When might a scoping study be appropriate for your post-graduate study?

A scoping study is a useful first step if you are undertaking a large-scale project such as a PhD or doctoral study. It can then be used as a basis for a more in-depth literature review as your project progresses. It provides an overview of the volume of published work in a topic area and may help to guide a subsequent more selective review.

Bibliometric analysis

This is an approach to mapping the trends in publication of literature in your area. Similar to a scoping study, the bibliometric analysis is an approach which is designed to describe and quantify trends in terms or concepts used in published papers (Papavasiliou et al. 2013). For example, it enables the reviewer to determine what research methodologies are popular in the published literature, which journals they are published in and the countries from which the research is published (Payne and Turner 2008). As with scoping studies, the bibliographic analysis does not incorporate all the steps of a formal literature review and does not include critical appraisal or detailed analysis and synthesis of the literature, but is an approach used to map volume and trends in the published literature on a particular topic.

Example of a bibliometric analysis

Papavasiliou et al. (2013) used a bibliographic analysis to map the trends in publications about continuous sedation prior to death. They found that publications had increased since the early 1990s and were published in a range of published literature in different journals but mostly from medical and health. The reviewers found differences in use of terminology and considerations of ethical practice.

When might a bibliometric analysis be appropriate for your post-graduate study?

You may consider using a bibliometric analysis as a component of your literature review in a doctoral or PhD study. In an in-depth study, you have the opportunity to explore many different methodological aspects of your study (we will discuss this in Chapter 3), and an examination of the publication and methodological trends in your research area can help you to set the context for your study.

In summary

There are many approaches to reviewing the literature and we have not attempted to present all of them in this chapter; methods of literature reviewing are continuously being developed and refined and any attempt to present a comprehensive overview would be quickly out of date. The methods we have presented are illustrative of the different types of approaches that are available.

While it is not necessary to follow a specified approach to your literature review within your post-graduate project, it is recommended that you consider all the common features of a review, which we have outlined on page 3 in Chapter 1. Most reviews share the common features of a research question, searching strategy, then appraisal of the research or other evidence identified which leads to a summary or interpretation of the results. Depending on the type of review you undertake, you will find that a different emphasis is placed on different features – for example, some reviews set clear criteria for quality assessment and do not include studies that do not meet these while others are more inclusive. These features are discussed throughout this book and it is important that you can justify the approach you undertake for your review.

If you do follow a specific approach to a literature review, we recommend that you access the relevant texts that describe this approach in full detail. As with all research methods, innovations and new ideas about possible methods are regularly published in academic journals and should be accessed if you decide to follow a particular approach.

The approach you take to your literature review will largely depend on the aim of your review and the type of research and other evidence that is relevant to it, as outlined in Table 2.1. Some literature reviews can be undertaken in a highly controlled way so that potential factors that might bias the outcomes are reduced and the review aims to provide a numerical (statistical) summary of the results: for example, a systematic review with meta-analysis. Other literature reviews do not aim to summarize the findings numerically but seek to describe and interpret the findings in order to provide a textual (thematic) summary of the results. Other approaches aim to incorporate both a numerical and thematic summary of the findings.

1. **Systematic review with meta-analysis**: a highly controlled approach with the aim of summarizing the findings of the included studies to a statistical form in order to test for significance
2. **Meta-aggregative review**: a controlled approach to the non-numerical summary of qualitative data which does not involve further interpretation of the studies
3. **Interpretative reviews of qualitative research**: a less controlled approach to the analysis and synthesis of qualitative studies which focusses on the re-interpretation of the studies included in the review

4. **Interpretative reviews of mixed methods**: a less controlled approach to the analysis and synthesis of qualitative, quantitative and other evidence which focusses on re-interpretation of the included studies
5. **Reviews which emphasize the role of pre-existing theory**: a theory-based approach for the analysis of literature where there are pre-defined concepts and theories
6. **Scoping study and bibliometric reviews**: overview approaches, which can be the forerunner to a larger review

Key points

- The methods for reviewing the literature have recently become more explicit, rigorous and are continuously developing.
- You may decide to follow an explicit method for your review.
- All methods share common features, which should be evident in all reviews.
- There are also some significant differences to the methods described.
- You need to be able to justify the approach you have taken when you write up your project or defend it in an oral examination.

3

What research and other evidence should I include in my literature review?

In this chapter we will discuss:
- *how empirical research will be relevant to your review*
- *how theories and concepts will be relevant to your review*
- *how research methods will be relevant to your review*

In Chapter 2, we discussed the different methods that have been developed for undertaking a literature review. In this chapter we will discuss the research and other evidence that you may include in your review. There is so much published information that you need to be able to recognize what is relevant for answering your review question. This will be guided by your research question, and your inclusion and exclusion criteria.

There are different types of literature that you are likely to engage with at different times in your review. When you are contemplating a literature review, it is often a review of the empirical research literature that

you may think of initially. By empirical literature we mean both qualitative and quantitative research in which data has been collected using
observational or experimental methods, providing evidence about what
has already been observed or known about the area you are studying.
This is because, in many cases, the empirical literature is best suited to
answering your research question, but this is not always the case and it
depends on your question and the inclusion and exclusion criteria you set.

However, you are also likely to discuss the research methods used
in the papers you have identified in order to help you select and defend
your choice of methods and to understand the research methods used by
others. You are also likely to consider the underlying theories and concepts in the papers you use in order to fully understand the background
to the papers you use and to help provide an explanatory framework
with which to interpret the literature you include in your review.

For this reason, your review might be divided into different
sections, often empirical, theoretical and methodological. The structure
will depend on the needs of your project. If your review is divided into
different sections, each will have its own focus and its own review question, and the literature you include within each section will depend on
the literature review question and the inclusion and exclusion criteria
you identify.

- The empirical literature is important as this enables you to bring
  together all the empirical research studies that have been undertaken
  which fit your inclusion and exclusion criteria.
- The theoretical literature is important in your review to ensure that
  your work, and the work of others, is understood and set within an
  appropriate theoretical framework. The data provided by your empirical literature review or your subsequent empirical study needs to be
  set in the context of other theories in order to make sense of and
  explain the results that you have.
- The methodological literature is important in your review as you are
  likely to refer to research undertaken in similar areas in order to help
  you to plan and justify the approaches you use in your own study. You
  also need to be able to understand the strengths and limitations of the
  methods used by others whose work you include in your review.

Given the large amount of information you are likely to come across, it
can be difficult to know where to start. Wallace and Wray (2011) present a system for categorizing evidence and identify four different types:
theory, research, practice, policy. This can be useful as it can prompt

you to consider the information you have against these categories and hence whether it is relevant to your review. Given the diversity of health and social care information, this assignment may not always be a straightforward task.

In general terms, Wallace and Wray's (2011) categories of theory and research are likely to be the types of literature most important to you in your review. This is because many review questions tend to be answered by data obtained from the systematic observation or experiments from the practice environment in health and social care, and associated concept and theories. In contrast, practice literature refers to discussion and accounts of practice and may not be assessed as rigorous evidence for inclusion in the results section of your review but may provide useful background information. Similarly, policies and guidelines are generally derived from research but in themselves may not constitute rigorous evidence for inclusion within a review. However, there is a caveat here; if your literature review question requires the review of policies or informal discussion or opinion, you would of course include this literature in your review.

Empirical, theoretical and methodological literature

In the majority of cases, literature review questions in health and social care are answered by a review of the empirical research literature, supported by a review of related theories and concepts and reference to methodological literature to justify your chosen approach (Finlayson and Dixon 2008). This principle applies to all reviews, whether a standalone review or one that is a pre-requisite to a larger study. The detail in which you are able to review the literature will depend on the scope of your study; it is particularly important if you are studying for a professional or taught doctorate or PhD but is also relevant to a research project which is a component of a MSc or master's award or a smaller-scale study.

Using empirical research, theories and reference to research methods in your review

For example, Preston (2004) undertook a PhD study to investigate the effectiveness of different approaches to managing malignant ascites, which are the build-up of fluid in the abdomen. The literature review was the pre-requisite to a larger empirical study and included a review of empirical, theoretical and methodological literature. Empirical research literature was reviewed to explore previous studies that had investigated different strategies for managing ascites so that the research was set in the context of what was already known about the topic. This literature review was informed by the theoretical literature, which was considered to establish what we know about the physiology of lymphoedema and why a particular strategy might be effective. In addition, the methodological literature was reviewed to examine possible ways in which the subsequent empirical study might be undertaken, by identifying methods that had been used in previous studies and the evaluation of those methods.

Empirical literature

Empirical research literature refers to studies where researchers use direct observation or experience to attempt to answer a research question. Sometimes the observations and experiences are collected in the natural environment and sometimes they are manipulated, for example, in an experiment. Data about observations and experience can be collected either qualitatively using textual descriptions or quantitatively using numerical measures, or sometimes using mixed methods where a combination of both qualitative and quantitative approaches are used. Both qualitative and quantitative data can be analysed thematically. Quantitative data can sometimes be analysed statistically.

There is a broad range of empirical research designs, from classic experiments (often referred to as randomized controlled trials, or RCTs) to variations on the classical experiment (for example cluster RCTs or quasi experiments), to surveys, and there is a wide variety of qualitative approaches. There is no one approach to empirical study that is 'better' than another but some are more suited to answering certain questions than others. Quantitative approaches are ideal for measuring that which is easily measurable and where direct comparisons are possible. Qualitative approaches are ideal for answering questions which seek in-depth meaning about a topic, or where an exploratory approach is required. Qualitative approaches are often undertaken where little is already known, and quantitative approaches are ideal for looking at relationships between concepts which are already well defined. It is beyond the scope of this book to explore all the major empirical methods but we strongly recommend that you are familiar with these methods before you commence your post-graduate studies. A research methods text-book should help facilitate this.

Inclusion of empirical literature in your literature review

The empirical literature that you include in your review will depend on the research question you are asking, but there are subtle differences in what you include depending on whether your review is supportive to a larger study or a standalone study in its own right.

- When the literature review is supportive and a pre-requisite to a larger empirical study, the empirical literature will generally be used to determine what has been done before and to identify the gap in the knowledge which will shape the research question for the larger study. Hence the aim of the review is to demonstrate the need and rationale for your subsequent empirical study.
- When the literature review is a standalone review, the empirical literature will generally be used to answer – or attempt to answer – the research question. Hence the aim of the review is to demonstrate what we know, rather than to demonstrate a gap in knowledge. However, this difference can be subtle as a standalone review can demonstrate that there is insufficient evidence to answer the review question.

The important point is that you recognize the role of the literature review and what it is helping you to achieve within your project.

Which empirical evidence is best for my literature review?

Some empirical studies will be better suited to addressing your literature review question than others. It is important that you can make a judge-ment about what studies will be most useful in answering your research question. There are practical and academic reasons to do this. Practi-cally, there is a lot of published information for almost every research question. Identifying the most appropriate evidence to include in your review is an important consideration so that you do not have to wade through a lot of inappropriate literature. Academically, given that cer-tain types of empirical research are going to be more relevant than oth-ers, it is important to identify what these are so that your search for relevant empirical research is focussed.

Different types of study designs are useful for answering different questions. Although RCTs are often used by Cochrane Collaboration reviewers, these reviews are usually focussed on answering questions about effectiveness and so these studies are appropriate. Even so, only RCTs that include sufficient information to calculate effect sizes can be included. For other literature review questions, other study designs are likely to be more relevant, and the type of study design that is most relevant will be determined by the literature review in question (Tucker and Roth 2005; Fielding 2010; Noyes 2010; Pearson 2010). The Joanna Briggs Institute (2014) argues that there should be a match between the method of the empirical research to be considered for the review and the review question.

It can therefore be useful to identify the types of study designs that are most likely to inform your literature review, so that you can search for these in the first instance. While prior identification of possible relevant study designs will not be definitive, it will help to guide you to what is likely to be appropriate for inclusion in your literature review in the first instance.

Considerations of hierarchies of evidence

You may come across the term 'hierarchy of evidence'. This term refers to the positivist tradition of ranking research and other evidence in terms of research designs which are most likely to eliminate bias. Bias is eliminated using strategies such as randomization and blinding, and those studies which are able to control for this are considered to be the least biased. Hierarchies of evidence are based on the principle that certain types of research designs will be less biased than others.

The most well-known hierarchy of evidence was developed by Sackett et al. (1996) in order to rank which research designs provide the strongest evidence for determining the effectiveness of a treatment or intervention. This hierarchy is based on the assumption that studies that provide a direct comparison of a treatment or intervention are the best way to determine effectiveness, that controlling for bias within studies is possible and that studies with the least bias will provide the strongest evidence. This hierarchy places systematic review of RCTs at the top, followed by RCTs, and qualitative studies near the bottom, because of the ability of RCTs to determine the effectiveness of treatments and interventions due to the rigour and degree of control that they have (Figure 2.1).

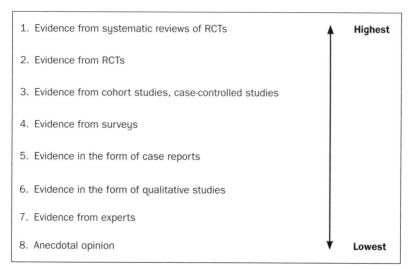

1. Evidence from systematic reviews of RCTs   **Highest**

2. Evidence from RCTs

3. Evidence from cohort studies, case-controlled studies

4. Evidence from surveys

5. Evidence in the form of case reports

6. Evidence in the form of qualitative studies

7. Evidence from experts

8. Anecdotal opinion   **Lowest**

Figure 2.1 Hierarchy of evidence for determining the effectiveness of a treatment or intervention

This hierarchy of evidence is one hierarchy but it is not the only hierarchy that may be relevant to your literature review. This hierarchy is *only* relevant for literature review questions that are concerned with measuring the effectiveness of interventions. Despite this, the hierarchy developed by Sackett et al. (1996) is sometimes oversimplified and referred to as 'the hierarchy of evidence' (Hoppe et al. 2009), implying that RCTs are always stronger than other studies in terms of the strength of evidence they provide. Given that different review questions will be best informed by different study designs, clearly there is no one 'hierarchy of evidence' that can be applied indiscriminately to all literature review questions.

Nor is there one type of research design that is always the most relevant to all literature review questions (Wall 2008; Denzin 2009; Merlin et al. 2009; Freshwater et al. 2010; Ford and Maher 2013).

Identifying which empirical research will be relevant for your review

To start at a very basic level, if your literature review question addresses an exploratory question about which little is known, you may seek other exploratory studies to help address the question. Qualitative studies are likely to be useful in this instance. If on the other hand, your literature review addresses a question about the relationship between different concepts that can be directly compared, then the literature that you include is likely to be that which has already analysed these relationships. Quantitative studies may be useful here. It is important to note that your final literature review is likely to include a broader range of literature than this brief summary might indicate, but it can be helpful to consider which literature you will be looking for in the first instance, to get your literature review started.

Before you undertake your empirical literature review, you should write a protocol or plan for your study. This will enable you to identify the literature that is relevant for your review. For example, researchers whose protocol for a systematic review is registered with the Cochrane Collaboration will consider and plan the type of literature they will seek in addressing their review question. If the question concerns the effectiveness of an intervention (for example, Cochrane Collaboration systematic reviews), reviewers are likely to indicate that they will be looking for RCTs, or reviews of RCTs, in the first instance, if these are available.

However, if your literature review question is investigating how social workers approach conversations about confidentiality in their practice, you would probably need to include a number of different research designs, and RCTs would probably not be relevant. In this case, you would be looking for research that explores the practice of social workers in a day-to-day context. This might include a range of qualitative and observational research designs from case studies involving interviews with practitioners and also interviews with their clients.

If you are exploring the impact of introducing smoke-free policies in a setting, you would be searching for literature that explores the views and attitudes and actions of people who live or work within that setting. This literature is likely to consist of exploratory interviews, focus groups and possibly questionnaires in addition to before and after studies that explore changes in rate of smoking.

So you can see that there is no one type of research design that is most appropriate for the different literature review questions mentioned above. The type of research design you need to include depends entirely on your research question.

Finding the appropriate 'hierarchy of evidence' for your study

Given that different literature review questions require different research designs to answer them, Noyes (2010) gives examples of alternative 'hierarchies' which may be appropriate for different literature review questions. Noyes (2010) argues that qualitative approaches can be used to answer more exploratory questions, such as when exploring patients' or clients' views and experiences of services and interventions. She emphasizes that, in this case, qualitative studies are likely to be more useful for describing patient or client experiences than quantitative studies, and this will be reflected in the literature identified in the search for relevant research.

Noyes (2010, p. 530) gives an example of a hierarchy of evidence that could help us understand client or patient experience. The hierarchy of 'views and experiences of interventions and services' is given in Figure 2.2.

Qualitative studies can also be used to examine many types of research question, such as why people behave in a certain way, what the needs of a group of people are, whether a treatment or intervention is feasible, whether a treatment or intervention can be improved, and so on.

Hierarchies of evidence can be a useful way to begin to consider which research methods are most relevant to your research question. However, they are a guide only and need to be considered flexibly – otherwise you risk omitting relevant literature from your review.

Some researchers would express caution at the concept of any attempt to rank evidence and would argue that it is problematic and over-simplistic and fails to engage with the complexities of the research

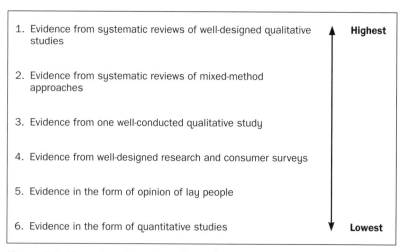

1. Evidence from systematic reviews of well-designed qualitative studies   **Highest**

2. Evidence from systematic reviews of mixed-method approaches

3. Evidence from one well-conducted qualitative study

4. Evidence from well-designed research and consumer surveys

5. Evidence in the form of opinion of lay people

6. Evidence in the form of quantitative studies   **Lowest**

Figure 2.2 Hierarchy of evidence for understanding the views and experiences of services users

you might come across. For example, these hierarchies place an order for certain studies but do not take into account how you should consider a study which is placed high in a hierarchy and is relevant to the review question but which has methodological flaws which affect its design and conduct.

Despite the complexities in the arguments, some research designs will be better suited to answering your review question than others and it is important to identify this when planning your literature review. Having a pre-determined idea of the type of research designs that you might include to answer your literature review question can be a useful way to commence your literature review, even if, on further engagement with the literature, you adapt and change your view of what research designs are most useful in answering your question.

Theoretical literature

If you only included empirical research in your project, you would have lots of interesting findings, taken from systematic observations and experiments, but you would not be able to generalize or transfer these findings beyond your study. Undertaking a review of the theoretical literature enables you to consider the theories, ideas and concepts that might shed light on the results of your empirical literature review. You can then use these theories to explain your results and findings and possibly generalize or transfer your findings to other contexts where this is appropriate. Without theories, you have lots of interesting findings but nothing to understand or interpret them with. When you include a review of the theoretical literature, you can incorporate your own findings with existing theories, ideas and concepts which may enable you to make some predictions and even develop the theories you have used. Theories are important as they provide a structure for your academic work, without which your ideas, even those gained from the empirical literature, are 'free floating' and cannot be easily applied to other contexts. In some literature reviews, you will be testing theories. When a theory is broken down into very small components, this might be referred to as a hypothesis, as in the example below.

- A theory is a well-established principle which explains some aspect of the natural world.
- A hypothesis is a specific and testable prediction about what you expect to happen.

In other literature reviews, you will be generating theories. Theories provide a link between the different research you bring together in your review and possible explanations for the ideas created. Without supporting theories, even something quite simple (as in the example below), it is hard to argue that your ideas are generalizable or transferable to another situation.

For example, Gøtzsche and Nielsen (2011) undertook a systematic review to test the theory that early detection of cancer saves lives. From this wider theory, they developed the hypothesis that early detection of breast cancer through mammography would also save lives. In their systematic review, the researchers collected and analysed the studies which had compared outcomes for women who had had mammography for the early detection of breast cancer, and those who had not, in order to test their hypothesis that screening can save lives. This review raised many methodological questions, for example whether it is acceptable to combine older and newer studies in a review and whether studies undertaken in different countries can be combined in the same analysis. All these questions added to the debate. However, the underlying hypothesis which was tested was whether the early detection of breast cancer can save lives. This was the basis for the systematic review. The results of this review contribute to the wider theoretical understanding about the role of early detection in the prevention and treatment of cancer.

So first it is important to be clear about what we mean by theory. The term theory is often used liberally in our everyday language. We might say 'in theory this should happen, but in practice . . .', indicating a gap between the ideal and the real world. For example, we also often refer to the 'theory component' of a health or social care course, which generally refers to a body of knowledge which is used to underpin the taught practical content.

There is also a more specific understanding of the term theory which we use in research and academic traditions, in which the term theory refers to connecting patterns and concepts so that predictions and explanations can be made about how things work and what might happen (Wallace and Wray 2011). The term theory used in this way is a way of connecting concepts so that our understanding of the world increases and generalizations can be made. This understanding – or theory – might be developed through patterns observed through either actual empirical observations or 'armchair' theorizing (Wallace and Wray 2011) and may incorporate abstract and general thinking. Some theories will be well supported by empirical evidence and others will not be and may be refuted. Substantial theories are important in any academic piece of work as they demonstrate an academic depth and rigour to the study and provide evidence that the researcher is able to apply the findings of the research to relevant contemporary theoretical concepts.

Not all theories have names. They are not necessarily erudite constructions. The theory or hypothesis mentioned in the example concerning whether early detection of cancer saves lives cannot be attributed to any one individual, although many scientists have worked to develop this theory. Other theories are attributable to certain individuals: for example, Einstein's theory of relativity.

Theory refers to our general and abstract understanding about a topic rather than that merely provided by the empirical literature. While the empirical literature explores what actually happens in the real world in a specific context, the theoretical literature draws these observations together in an attempt to explain aspects of the social or physical world, in order to make predictions about what is likely to happen. Empirical studies may be guided implicitly or explicitly by theoretical constructs. Some empirical studies aim explicitly to test competing theories, and all use theories to interpret their findings. Theories are essential to the work of researchers as they provide an explanatory framework through which the results of empirical research can be interpreted and provide a way of generalizing or transferring the results.

Before you can explore possible theories that you may include in your literature review, you need to be clear about the exact terms and concepts you are referring to.

Defining the concepts used in your literature review

When you are doing a literature review, it is fundamental to your emerging study that you are familiar with the body of knowledge that underpins your topic and that you define the terms and concepts you are using in your review. These will usually be the terms and concepts that are stated in your literature review question but there might be other terms you need to explore and clarify. So, for example, if your literature review concerns the role played by spirituality for those using a psychodynamic approach to counselling (we have deliberately chosen this question as it is a complex example), you would need to define the concepts of spirituality and psychodynamic counselling, which in itself would be challenging.

Exploration of the concepts used will usually involve a comparison of the different ways in which they have been used in the existing literature. You might undertake a concept analysis or scoping study to do this. Once you have reviewed the use of the concept, you need to commit to one understanding of the concept, even if the choice of definition you use feels somewhat arbitrary. You may consider that the concepts you use are clear and do not require further definition or clarification; however, it is essential to clarify their meaning and the conceptual underpinnings so that you can use them within your literature review.

Inclusion of theoretical literature in your literature review

During your post-graduate study, you are encouraged to identify theories and concepts that are relevant to your thesis as a whole. It is important to recognize what is a theory and what is not, referring back to the work of Wallace and Wray (2011) and to distinguish theories from the empirical findings.

Theories are likely to be explored initially in a background section of your literature review and returned to again once you have analysed your data in the discussion. This is the standard format for most literature reviews and empirical studies. However, if you are using qualitative methods such as grounded theory, your examination of theory will often be made once you have commenced the collection and analysis of your data rather than be identified at the beginning of the study. This is because when you undertake this type of exploratory study, you are generally seeking to generate theory rather than to test it so it is unusual to commence the study with explicit reference to theory. This is in order not to lead the data analysis and to keep an open mind about the emerging results of the study. Instead, reference to relevant theory will emerge as the analysis progresses. However, you need to be aware of potential implicit theoretical concepts that you may hold as these may become a source of bias in your analysis.

- When your literature review is supportive and a pre-requisite to a larger empirical study, relevant theories will be identified in the supporting literature review and often referred to in the analysis and interpretation of empirical data. There are some exceptions to this: for example, if you are undertaking a study as previously explained, perhaps a grounded theory study, and are developing your own theory, in which case you would avoid seeking out established theory prior to undertaking your own study.

- When your literature review is a standalone literature review, relevant theories will often be explored in the introduction and then referred to in the analysis and interpretations of the literature reviewed.

Searching for relevant theories

Searching for relevant theories can be a complex process, which we will discuss in detail in Chapter 4. Some theories are searchable by name; others are more elusive. Theories will often be identified through wide reading and knowledge of the key texts and researchers in your area. The amount of theoretical literature available can be very large and may vary in quality and scope.

Understanding competing theories

It is likely that you will find one or more competing theories about the topic you are studying. Theories come in and out of fashion and are adapted as we gain understanding through empirical observation.

In physics, there are mainline theories which many people might assume are firmly established. Yet even these are often refined. The ongoing search for a 'Grand Unified Theory', which could explain everything, would probably change any theories we currently have. Therefore no theory is fixed in stone.

Some theories will be robust and supported by strong empirical evidence while others will be less well supported and may be rejected. Further empirical evidence may enhance or decrease support for a theory and theoretical development. Often empirical research will test out, refine and develop new theories. Some theories can be no more than a hunch or an idea. For example, one very early theory that 'the world is flat' dominated the thinking of many early civilizations until advancements in science and travel led to its revision.

Theories develop as our knowledge develops. In health and social care, this is usually from the advancement of knowledge through empirical studies. So for example, there is the very well-known and established theory that smoking causes lung cancer. Most people would accept now that the possibility that this theory will be rejected is very small. However, it was the increase in empirical studies exploring the link between tobacco and lung cancer in the 1950s and 1960s that supported the development of this causal theory.

It is common to find theories that compete with each other. Take, for example, the theory of behaviour change, as described by Prochaska et al. (1994). This theory states that people work through a series of pre-defined stages during the process of behaviour change, for example in smoking cessation (Prochaska et al. (1994)), and was popular at the start of the twenty-first century. In contrast, West developed a competing theory that many people do not work through a series of stages in order to change a behaviour but instead can have an overnight decision to break a habit (West 2006).

From the examples given above, you can see that incorporating theories into your review can be a complex process. Relevant theories might be hard to find and not easy to search for. They may not be as easily identified as other types of literature, as we shall explore in Chapter 4. You might perceive that you have identified them by chance through background reading, and some theoretical positions might only be implicitly stated in empirical papers. You are likely to encounter many possible theories including those which compete with one another.

Example of how researchers used theories to support the design of a quantitative study

Lindson (2012) undertook a PhD study in which she compared those who gave up smoking abruptly as a means of smoking cessation with those who gave up by gradually reducing their smoking. A gradual reduction in smoking is regarded by many people as an intuitive approach to smoking cessation. This intuitive hunch is supported by theorists such as Balfour and Fagerstrom (1996), who suggest that abrupt abstinence can heighten the experience of withdrawal symptoms and may be enough to drive an individual to return to smoking; a gradual reduction should reduce the impact of this. Lindson (2012) carried out a Cochrane Collaboration review as a pre-requisite to a larger empirical study to test this theory, whether those who reduced their smoking prior to quitting produced similar quit rates to those who gave up smoking abruptly.

Extract from Lindson's research study (2012, p. 8)

Some withdrawal symptoms commonly experienced as a result of the nicotine abstinence syndrome are irritability, restlessness, difficulty concentrating, impaired task performance, anxiety, hunger, weight gain, sleep disturbance, cravings and drowsiness . . . . Therefore it has been suggested that many smokers continue smoking to avoid these negative effects of abstinence (Balfour and Fagerstrom 1996) and indicate that reduction in smoking might be a viable alternative as a smoking cessation approach.

The results of the review indicated a similar smoking cessation rate in those who gave up abruptly and those who gradually reduced their smoking. The results were discussed in the light of Balfour and Fagerstrom's (1996) theory.

Example of how researchers used theories to provide context for a qualitative study

Taylor (2012) undertook a PhD study to investigate the experiences of intimacy and sexuality for people living with a life-limiting illness. Taylor used the theories of Heidegger not only to provide a rationale and guide for her phenomenological approach (Taylor and de Vocht, 2011), but also to provide a theoretical underpinning for her analysis. Heidegger's (1962, p. 158) theory of 'solicitude' [*Fürsorge*], which he used to describe caring for another, enhanced Taylor's understanding of what it means for partners who take on a caring role.

Extract from Taylor's research study (2012, p. 108)

[S]olicitude has two extreme possibilities. It can, as it were, take away 'care' from the Other and put itself in his position in concern: it can leap in for him. This kind of solicitude takes over for the Other that which he is to concern himself. The Other is thus thrown out of his own position . . . In such solicitude the Other can become one who is dominated and dependent, even if this domination is a tacit one and remains hidden from him . . . In contrast to this, there is also the possibility of a kind of solicitude which does not so much leap in for the Other as leap ahead of him (*ihm vorausspringt*) in his existentiell [sic] potentiality-for-being, not in order to take away his 'care' but rather to give it back to him authentically as such for the first time.

Research has shown that both men (Gilbert et al. 2009) and women (Gilbert et al. 2009; Hawkins et al. 2009) who care for their sick partners can re-position them as a 'child', and cease to view them as a sexual partner. However, Taylor's (2015) research found that performing intimate caring tasks did not necessary prevent intimacy and sexual expression within couples' relationships. Heidegger's (1962) theory of solicitude helped Taylor (2015) to understand the nuances in the care that partners provide. She gives the example of one partner of a profoundly disabled man who had provided her husband's care for him ('leap in caring'). When providing intimate care, this partner no longer saw her husband in a sexual way, and was unable to respond to his request for a kiss. In Heidegger's (1962, p. 158) words, he was 'thrown out of his own position' as her lover during intimate care.

Puzzled by the differences in other couples' experiences, Taylor (2015) realized that 'leap in caring' is not simply a matter of performing physical tasks for one's partner, but involves moving from a position of mutual equality to one of 'carer' and 'cared for' in their emotional relationship. Using Heidegger's (1962) theory to support this analysis, Taylor (2015) concluded that, regardless of whether the care that is provided is physically intimate, it is changes to the equality in couples' relationships that impacts upon their sexual and intimate relationship.

These two examples illustrate how you might incorporate theories in your project and use them to develop your ideas and arguments. The theories you use will require a judgement about their relevance. It is not always possible to get a complete or exhaustive picture of all the potentially relevant theories that are associated with your research question or topic. Any topic could be informed by many different theories. You would usually engage with the theories that are relevant to your academic discipline. So, for example, if your project is situated within psychology, you would be likely to refer to psychological theories rather than sociological theories even though some sociological theories might have clear relevance to your work.

If you are doing a PhD or doctoral-level study, your engagement with theories and concepts will be more extensive than for those studying at master's level. However, at master's level you would usually be expected to identify relevant theories which provide an explanatory framework for your project in a section of your literature review and to refer back to them in the discussion section of your dissertation. It is useful to explore some of the relevant theories so that you have an anchor upon which to develop your ideas as your study progresses. It is also important that you can discuss and critique the theoretical ideas you encounter. You need to be able to recognize which theories will be relevant to your literature review and that you can distinguish them from more general background information. It is also important that you can identify the extent to which the theories are supported by empirical literature and how relevant they are to your literature review.

Methodological literature

Methodological literature refers to those papers (or aspects of papers) that investigate or describe research methods and practices. You might come across a paper that focusses solely on the discussion of methods used in a study reported elsewhere or you might find a detailed discussion of methods used within a study which also reports the findings of the empirical research. Methodological literature is important in many ways when you are writing a literature review.

You will get a feel for the type of research that has been carried out in your area and this may enable you to do a more focussed or refined search for further research of this kind. This might help with your search strategy, which we will discuss in Chapter 4. Focussing on the methodological aspects of a study will help you to understand and critically evaluate the research methods used by other researchers whose work you are using and critiquing in your review. We will discuss this further in Chapters 5 and 6.

Most importantly, however, the examination of the methods used in empirical studies might also help you select and justify what methods to use for your own study. Reviewing the methods of published research can help you establish and decide upon your own method for your research – be it a standalone literature review or a larger empirical study if appropriate.

- When the literature review is supportive and a pre-requisite to a larger empirical study, methodological literature may be used to identify suitable methods for the empirical study. You can critique the methods used in the papers you identify for your review in order to help you identify appropriate research methods.

- When the literature review is a standalone one the methodological literature can be used to justify your approach taken to your literature review method. You may also use the methodological literature to comment on the research approaches used in the literature you include in your review.

For example, when we were writing this book, much scrutiny was given to the methods used by those who had undertaken various types of literature reviews. We have scrutinized the methods sections of research papers and contacted researchers to get a better insight as to why they used the methods they reported. This focus on the way different researchers used the literature review methods enabled us to consider the consistency with which different approaches were used and to build up a picture of the common features occurring in most literature reviews. You can use the methodological literature to justify overarching approaches, such as a literature review method, or individual methods within a research design, such as approaches to interviewing.

Inclusion of methodological literature in your literature review

If your literature review is a pre-requisite to a larger empirical study, you can refer to the existing research methods literature to develop the appropriate research methods for your own study. By the time you have searched for literature in your research area, you will have a body of empirical material documenting the studies that are relevant to your research. When you read the empirical studies related to your own research area, it is useful to consider more than just the findings from the empirical results of the study. In addition to using these studies to inform your knowledge about previous work that has been undertaken, you can use this literature to identify *how* previous research has been undertaken and how researchers have evaluated their use of these methods. You can examine the details of the methods and evaluations of these methods used by the researcher to help you refine the method for your own study. You can then refer to and/or review these methods and take notice of their limitations to help you develop your own methods for your empirical study.

To start with, you are likely to examine the research methods used in the empirical research you have already identified as relevant to your research area, but it might also be useful to examine research methods of studies which are not directly related to your review or subsequent empirical study but where the methods might be transferable. Depending on how you use the empirical literature, some additional searches related to methods may be required, especially if you draw on studies that you are not using in your empirical literature review.

Using methodological literature to shape the design of your study

Papers identified in a literature review can help you shape and design the research methods you use in your study. You are most likely to do this if your literature review is 'supportive' to a larger study in which you are developing methods to use in your empirical study. However, if your literature review is a standalone review you will need to justify the approach you have chosen to undertake your own literature review.

> Some researchers might put the discussion of methodological aspects of the research in the methodology section of their thesis. Others might put it in the literature review section. It is up to individual researchers to decide where this section best fits into their work but the focus needs to be clear that the review of empirical literature is undertaken in order to assess the methods used in order to inform the methods used in your own study.

We will use some examples from the literature review section of three reviews to illustrate how the methodological literature has been used to inform the development of research methods for a larger empirical study.

Example of how researchers used the methodological literature to justify the use of interviews in their study

Methodological literature can be used to identify methods which have been used by others who have undertaken research in a similar area to your own study. These methods can then be considered to see if they are suitable and relevant methods that might help you address your research question.

For example, a research study was carried out in Switzerland, a country where assisted suicide is legal under certain circumstances. Assisted suicide refers to the practice of patients taking a prescribed concoction of drugs to end their life (physician- or volunteer-assisted suicide). Researchers searched for previously published research and identified in the literature review that, unsurprisingly, the majority of the existing research was based upon survey design. While the surveys went some way in describing the experiences, there was no depth to the findings, as might be expected from such an approach. The benefits of using surveys were that they did not expose either the researcher or family member to difficult conversations and could be conducted alone and with anonymity. The disadvantage of using surveys was that the depth of understanding of experience remained largely unexplored. It might seem that interviews with bereaved families following such a traumatic experience would be very sensitive and difficult to conduct and that this would prohibit their use in such research. Yet without them, the lived experiences of family members and health care staff remain unexplored.

In order to address this, a search for further empirical literature was carried out to identify research studies in which interviews had been conducted with family members and healthcare staff following particularly sensitive and difficult bereavements. The literature showed that even in difficult circumstances, interviews had been conducted and that these were possible and acceptable to all of those involved.

This example illustrates how the empirical literature enabled the researcher to identify and justify appropriate research methods for a proposed study. Use of the methodological literature in this example not only helped the researcher to identify a gap in the research regarding a lack of in-depth understanding of experience but also helped her to identify appropriate ways in which a sensitive situation might be discussed using interviews, and she was able to justify a design for an empirical study using a grounded theory approach. Without referring to the experience of other researchers' use of interviews in sensitive situations, this would have been less easy to justify.

Example of how researchers used the methodological literature to identify a method of measurement in their study

Methodological literature can be used to identify methods of undertaking an intervention to be used in a study and how a certain type of measurement can be obtained.

For example, a research study was undertaken to determine the optimum management in clinical practice of the build-up of ascites in patients with a malignancy. The management of ascites refers to how we help patients with large volumes of fluid which can build up in the peritoneal (abdominal) cavity. This research was undertaken to explore how this process could be managed most effectively and acceptably for the patient. A vital part of the research was the measurement of pressure in the intra-peritoneal cavity. It was important to determine the best way of measuring this. A literature review had been conducted to identify papers which recorded ways of measuring intra-abdominal pressure. The review identified that the main method applied had been to use an approximation for abdominal pressure rather than to measure it directly. In order to do this, the patient had been given pressure-sensitive telemetry pills to swallow and an approximation of abdominal pressure had been made from the stomach. However, this process is not an exact simulation for abdominal ascites as the stomach is a muscular structure which would also be undergoing constriction itself, which could result in a change of pressure. The researcher felt that this approach was sub-optimal and that direct measurement, in which the peritoneal cavity was accessed through a drainage tube, was preferable. This should have been possible using a narrow pressure transducer, which could be fed down the tube used to drain the ascites. However, what was unknown was the pressure range that the pressure transducer needed to be sensitive to. A subsequent review of the literature was undertaken in order to estimate upper and lower pressure ranges from indirect measurements. As a result, an upper limit was set and a transducer purchased which was sensitive enough to show changes in pressure slightly beyond this upper limit (Preston 2004).

This example illustrates how the methodological literature can be used for guidance about how to obtain measurements that are required in a research project. It also illustrates how the knowledge and understanding obtained by previous researchers can enhance the method of future studies.

Example of how researchers used the methodological literature to develop strategies for recruitment in their study

Methodological literature can be used to determine the most effective ways to recruit participants into a study.

For example, a research study was undertaken to investigate the experience of patients who belonged to a 'hard to reach' group and hence were not easy to identify or subsequently to recruit. Recruitment is a major issue for most research studies, often with only 50 per cent of studies recruiting to target (Treweek et al. 2013). Therefore the recruitment problem is intensified for 'hard to reach' populations, such as people with alcohol-related cirrhosis. This can be due to the stigma related to the diagnosis or due to problems identifying and accessing potential participants because of the organization of care service where, for example, not all participants come to a set clinic on a given day. In order to address these recruitment difficulties, researchers for this study reviewed the literature to identify ways in which researchers in published studies had tackled the difficulty in recruitment of 'hard to reach' groups, such as the homeless. They were able to identify a range of strategies that helped to optimize recruitment.

These examples illustrate how the scrutiny of the methods used by other researchers can help inform the choice you make about methodological decisions in your own project. These should be written up when you discuss the research methods you selected in your study. You can discuss the ways in which you referred to the work of others, research methods you found helpful and those you chose not to use.

In summary

It is important to remember to set your project within the existing empirical, theoretical and methodological work that has been undertaken in your area. Your project will not reach its full potential until you can demonstrate how your review relates to other work in the area. The phrase 'standing on the shoulders of giants' is applicable here.

At all levels of study, your engagement with the empirical research literature is likely to be the main emphasis of your literature review. Drawing on the existing empirical work that informs the area is a central feature of undertaking a literature review. However, it is also important to draw on the work of others who have engaged with theories, ideas and concepts that are related to your area and the methods that others have used in their studies, in order to help you develop your methods for your review and subsequent empirical study where applicable.

If you are doing a PhD or doctoral-level study, your review of the empirical, theoretical and methodological literature will be more extensive than for those studying at master's level, and you need to make a judgement, in collaboration with your supervisor, about the level of engagement which is appropriate for your study.

In the next chapter, we will discuss how you can search for empirical, theoretical and methodological literature.

Key points

- In all post-graduate study, it is important to set your work within the context of others.
- This includes review of theories and methods in addition to the empirical literature.
- Empirical literature will enable you to discuss the existing research.
- Theoretical literature will enable you to explore theories, concepts and ideas.
- Methodological literature will enable you to explore possible research methods to inform your study.

4

How do I search for relevant literature?

In this chapter we will discuss:
- *why a comprehensive search strategy is important*
- *when you might use different approaches to searching*
- *how to search electronic databases*
- *how to employ additional search strategies*

In this chapter we will explore how you search for the different types of literature that you may include in your review. We will discuss this with reference to searching for empirical, theoretical and methodological literature.

When you identify your question for your literature review, you will identify inclusion and exclusion criteria which will enable you to focus your search. Your search will be directed by your review question and the criteria for inclusion you set.

How comprehensive does my search need to be?

At first, you might think that you need to find every possible piece of literature that is relevant to your review. In reality, you need to think carefully about the scope of your review so that you move quickly from discussion of the very general to the specific research and other evidence that is relevant to your project. You are unlikely to have the time or the word count in your thesis to discuss more general issues related to your project and if you do, this is likely to be at the expense of the more detailed examination of research and other evidence that is directly relevant to your study. Focussing in on the literature that is specifically relevant to your project requires a judgement as you clearly need to set the context of your study. The important point to remember is that you are likely to be limited by a word count and you cannot afford to 'waste' words on generic matters relating to your topic; you need to focus on the specific area you are researching as soon as possible. You are likely to include more background information in an introduction. We will discuss this further in Chapter 8 when we consider the art and science of writing up a literature review.

Comprehensive searching

Once you have established the specific focus of your review, your review question and inclusion and exclusion criteria, your search for relevant literature that meet these criteria will usually be comprehensive.

For example, Mason (2014) undertook a PhD study in which he explored the experiences of older drug users in their drug-taking patterns and their interactions with healthcare professionals. His literature review was therefore a pre-requisite to his larger empirical study. The main focus of Mason's literature review was empirical research that had been undertaken by previous researchers who had investigated the experiences of older drug users and their interactions with healthcare professionals. For this section of the literature review, the researcher required a comprehensive search as it was essential that Mason identified all the studies that had previously been undertaken which related directly to his study focus; that is, which met his inclusion criteria. Any omissions might have led to a gap in his review and hence incomplete conclusions could have been drawn which could have affected his subsequent empirical study.

This type of comprehensive approach to literature searching is sometimes referred to as an 'exhaustive' approach. In this type of search, it is important that you identify all relevant research or other evidence so that your review is comprehensive and does not omit significant work in the area, as discussed in Chapter 1. This is the approach advocated by the Cochrane Collaboration, and it requires that researchers should obtain all available empirical evidence that addresses the literature review (or systematic review) question. Specific advice in the Cochrane *Handbook* is that literature reviewers should

> *attempt to collate all empirical evidence that fits pre-existing eligibility criteria in order to answer a specific research question. It uses explicit, systematic methods that are selected with a view to minimising bias, thus providing more reliable findings from which conclusions can be drawn and decisions made.*
>
> (Higgins and Green 2011)

We suggest that, where possible, you endeavour to undertake an exhaustive or comprehensive search for the research and other evidence that address your review question and that meet your inclusion and exclusion criteria (Noblit and Hare 1988; Barosso et al. 2003; Dixon-Woods et al. 2005; Walsh and Downe 2005). Where an exhaustive search is not feasible, you should undertake as comprehensive a search as is reasonable within the limitations of your resources for your project. This is because, in your literature review, you are seeking to find every relevant piece of literature in order to avoid 'cherry picking' evidence and omitting vital research, whose omission might bias or affect the review. Your aim is to identify all the available literature which might contribute to answering the literature review question.

This involves explicit planning of the exact focus of the review, key terms and synonyms and identifying appropriate databases. The literature search usually extends beyond a database search and includes other strategies for identifying appropriate literature – such as reference list searching, citation tracking and contacting key researchers – so that no stone is left unturned in the search for literature, including that which is unpublished. We discuss additional strategies for identifying literature later in this chapter.

Although your search should usually be comprehensive, it is important to note that not everything will be incorporated into the results of your review. Much of the research and other evidence you identify will be filtered out by inclusion and exclusion criteria so that everything you include is directly relevant to your review. These inclusion and exclusion criteria will include considerations of relevance, quality or appropriateness of research method and will be justified with a clear rationale, which we will discuss later in this chapter. Sometimes the inclusion criteria will specify particular research methods for inclusion in the study. For example, in Cochrane Collaboration reviews of effectiveness, the review protocols may specify that only randomized controlled trials (RCTs) are included in the review, as these are considered to be the best evidence in this type of review. In addition, other quality criteria are sometimes applied so that only the very 'best available' evidence is included. For example, you may decide to include only interview-based studies rather than questionnaires if your review is of a particularly sensitive topic and you do not feel that data from questionnaires will have sufficient depth to be relevant. This will depend on the individual review concerned, and judgement is made by the reviewers as to the inclusion and exclusion criteria set.

Selective or purposive searching

The alternative to a fully comprehensive search for literature is a selective or purposive search. In this approach, researchers do not seek to identify all literature but search for a selection of literature that meets the needs of the review. This approach may be undertaken in certain large-scale qualitative and mixed-method reviews where the literature review is a standalone study and where the aim of the review is interpretative rather than aggregative or summative. In this case, reviewers often aim to develop concepts or to capture the main themes arising in a body of literature and cease searching when new literature does not add to conceptual clarity, understanding or knowledge development (Noblit and Hare 1988; Dixon-Woods et al. 2005; Thomas and Harden 2008; Hannes and Macaitis 2012; Finfgeld-Connett and Johnson 2013).

For example, in their Cochrane Collaboration qualitative systematic review of barriers and facilitators to the implementation of lay health workers to improve access to maternal and child health, Glenton et al. (2013) used a purposive or selective approach to the literature included in their study. They extracted data from the results of the included qualitative studies. Glenton et al. (2013) report that it is not always practical to analyse large amounts of qualitative research in the depth required in order to avoid a simplistic overview and they describe how too many studies can threaten the quality of data analysis.

The appropriateness of taking a selective or purposive approach to literature searching and sampling for an empirical qualitative or mixed-method literature review is widely debated among researchers.

Atkins et al. (2008) challenged the logic behind identifying a purposive sample; that is, it is not possible to know that additional unidentified literature will not add to the existing theme or clarity to existing concepts. For example, themes might seem to be saturated after the analysis of 20 papers, but the 21st paper might add a new dimension which would remain unidentified if the search had ceased at 20 papers.

For the purposes of this book, we argue that purposive or selective searching should not be undertaken by those doing a literature review without a strong rationale. It is generally restricted to those undertaking a large-scale standalone qualitative or mixed-method review who have made a judgement that a comprehensive search is not appropriate in that particular context. This is a judgement that needs to be defended when writing up the method undertaken for the review or possibly in the oral examination.

Selective or purposive searching may be relevant when you are searching for additional methodological and theoretical literature to supplement the literature you have already identified in your comprehensive search. Searching for theories can be a complex process, even if you commence your project with a clear idea of the theories you will be referring to in your work. You are unlikely to be required to identify all the possible theories that might relate to your project – unless the specific demands of your project require this. You are expected to identify relevant theories that can help you to explain the data that you analyse in your review. The process of searching for theories is likely to be iterative as different theories may be explored and reviewed for the contribution they make to the understanding of the research question. Similarly, the search for methodological literature is not, and does not need to be comprehensive, as researchers are looking for examples and justification for the approaches taken to research design. The aim of referring to the supporting methodological literature is to provide examples and justification for the research methods you have chosen rather than to provide a comprehensive discussion of all possible appropriate methods.

For example, Mason (2014) justified his approach of in-depth interviews to investigate the experiences of older people who used illicit drugs by referring to a selection of previous research in which this research method had been used to investigate the habits of similar 'hard to reach' groups. He used the methods undertaken by previous researchers, including strategies to contact and recruit potential participants, to inform the design of his study. He also used these research studies to search for theories which might help him understand the ongoing data analysis from his empirical study.

Additional searches

Whichever strategy you employ for the search for research and other evidence, you are likely to undertake supplementary searches for theoretical and methodological literature as the needs of your project demand (Table 4.1). These searches will be additional to the comprehensive search you are likely to have undertaken. These searches might also 'snowball' from the existing literature identified from your comprehensive search (Greenhalgh and Peacock 2005), for example from reading lists of identified studies.

The search strategy

For some literature reviews, for example Cochrane Collaboration reviews, the search strategy is completely pre-defined. The search strategy might be tested in advance but once it is established, it is the one that is used and often formally updated every 3–5 years. In other reviews, the search strategy may evolve as the project proceeds in a more iterative manner. Chapman et al. (2009) observe that searching is also often conducted in several phases and is not necessarily a linear process. The search strategy may not be pre-defined in specific detail but emerges as the literature is identified, and investigation of one area of literature might lead to exploration of further literature. Finfgeld-Connett and Johnson (2013) argue that searching is not a linear or 'one-off' process and cannot be determined accurately at the start of the project. In fact those proposing the approach sometimes argue that prior thinking and pre-definition of all terms may preclude creativity and thinking about the concepts and may inhibit their development. Therefore, in some projects, you may return to the databases for additional searches when the need becomes apparent as you progress with your project.

Table 4.1 How inclusive does my literature search need to be?

	Research and other evidence that meet your inclusion and exclusion criteria	Supporting theoretical literature	Supporting methodological literature
Your main project is an empirical study. The literature review is a **supportive literature review**.	You should usually aim to include *all* empirical research and other evidence which meets your inclusion and exclusion criteria for your literature review question.	You should aim to discuss the main theories, concepts and ideas that relate to your research question in some detail.	You should aim to refer to the methods used by other researchers who have researched similar areas or participant groups to justify the methods you adopt for your study.
Your main project is a literature review from which you hope to answer a research question. We will refer to this as a **standalone literature review**.			If your main project is a literature review, you are likely to include a rationale for the approach to the literature review you have chosen (for example, systematic review, meta-ethnography).

Developing a search strategy

Once you have established the purpose of your literature review and your approach to searching, you need to develop a search strategy that is appropriate to the requirements of your project and which will enable you to identify and locate the most relevant range of published and unpublished material (where relevant) to answer your research question.

Specialist librarian input

You are strongly advised to consult an academic librarian to assist you with developing your search strategy. Your university, hospital library or professional body may be able to assist you in seeking advice from a specialist librarian. However, remember that you will be required to defend your approach to searching either in your written thesis or in an oral examination, and you should not delegate the task of searching to a third party. It is your project and you need to keep control of this process. When you consult a specialist librarian, ensure that they are aware that you are searching for a literature review and that you are looking for everything that addresses your question in the first instance (unless you have made a conscious decision not to do this, as discussed earlier in this chapter), rather than a more refined and manageable list of possible references. The important point to remember is that there is a difference between writing an essay, where you are interested in relevant references on your topic, and writing a literature review, where you are interested in all the references on your topic. Specialist librarians are trained to guide researchers and professionals towards both of these options and you therefore need to be specific about the needs of your individual project when discussing your search strategy.

Defining key terms

In order to search for research and other evidence about your literature review question, the first step is to identify the key terms under which research and other evidence may be identified in an electronic database and with which you would recognize the potentially relevant titles and abstracts stored in a database. The reason behind identifying key terms is that when journal articles are entered onto a database, they are identified by the key terms. Journal articles can then be identified when the same key terms are entered onto a database and the relevant articles will be retrieved.

Key terms are the important words or ideas in your literature review question which should be included in an article you are looking for, in order for it to be relevant to you. Key terms are either identified by you as the researcher or they can be identified from a pre-prepared list – for example, as subject headings, MeSH (medical subject headings) terms or thesaurus terms – which you will find listed within the database. We will discuss both of these options later in this chapter. Every database works slightly differently and it is important to become familiar with the database you are using so that you can search using your own key terms or those pre-identified in the subject headings (or equivalent).

Key terms and synonyms

In addition to key terms, it is also necessary to identify as many synonyms, or words that mean the same thing as the key term, as possible. This maximizes your chances of finding research and other evidence that may use different terminology but which none the less is relevant to your literature review. It is important that your key terms and synonyms should be as extensive and comprehensive as possible, while not deviating too far from the original term for which you are searching. For example, Clark et al. (2013) report using over a hundred key terms. Langenhoff and Schoones (2011) report using over a thousand combinations of key terms. Key terms can be identified by a simple 'brainstorm' of relevant phrases that might be used in connection with your topic, including words no longer currently used. Ideas for key terms can also be identified from papers which you have already, or might be obtained using simple Google searches which link you to other general information on your review question.

Care and consideration are needed when identifying key terms. For example, the key term 'qualitative' will not necessarily access all qualitative research, as many databases have only recognized this term as a key term in recent years (Noyes and Popay 2007). Furthermore, the term 'qualitative' is a broad term and is likely to identify papers unrelated to qualitative research.

Tools to assist the development of key terms

In addition to the strategies mentioned above for the identification of key terms, various tools or acronyms have been developed in order to facilitate the identification of an appropriate range of key terms and synonyms. One of the most well known is the PICO (Population, Intervention, Comparison, Outcome) tool, which has become widely used to enable researchers to define their research question and hence their search strategy. PICO has been adopted by the Cochrane Collaboration (Cooke et al. 2012) as a guide to both the formulation of the research question and the identification of key terms and synonyms. The origins of the PICO tool can be traced back to the early discussion about evidence-based practice (Richardson 1998) and the importance of asking a clearly focussed question with clearly defined elements.

Richardson (1998) identified that good clinical questions generally contain three or four well-defined elements and these have become the basis of the PICO acronym. Using this acronym as a trigger, researchers are encouraged to identify a key term and relevant alternative terms or synonyms for the population, intervention, comparison and outcomes appropriate to their literature review question. The version of PICO described above has its origins in the quantitative domain, with reference to interventions and comparisons. Alternative tools and acronyms have been developed which are considered to be more appropriate for literature review questions which are more qualitative. Fineout-Overholt and Johnston (2005) discuss the adaptation of the PICO tool for qualitative research questions: Population, Issue, Context, Outcome. In this version, some of the 'quantitative' terms used in the original PICO version have been replaced with 'qualitative' terms: namely, intervention is replaced by issue and comparison is replaced by context.

Another tool or acronym is SPICE: Setting, Population, Intervention, Comparison, Evaluation. With this tool, Cooke et al. (2012) recognize the evaluative nature of qualitative research, with the addition of evaluation; however, the quantitative origins of the tool are still evident as the focus is on intervention and comparison. Another more qualitative tool is SPIDER: Sample, Phenomena of Interest, Design, Evaluation, Research type. In this tool, population is replaced by sample (Cooke et al. 2012) (Table 4.2).

Which tool or acronym should I use?

The purpose of these acronyms is to enhance the identification of key terms and synonyms that will lead you to the most relevant references for the literature review. The aim is that using a tool will trigger the identification of key terms and synonyms that might remain otherwise unidentified. Thus use of the tool should trigger the most comprehensive search for literature.

Each of the different tools focusses on different elements of the research question and hence will have a different emphasis on the subsequent search strategy. In order to find out how effective these tools or acronyms are at triggering researchers to identify the most appropriate key terms and synonyms, a formal evaluation of each would be required. When you decide to use one of these tools, it is useful to consider the evaluations that have been carried out. It is beyond the scope of this book to review the literature for tools and acronyms and their evaluations; however, two such evaluations of these tools have been identified.

Table 4.2   Different tools for identifying key terms

PICOT – quantitative (Higgins and Green 2011)
- **P**opulation
- **I**ntervention
- **C**omparison
- **O**utcome
- **T**ime (not always included)

PICOT – qualitative (Fineout-Overholt and Johnston 2005)
- **P**opulation
- **I**ssue
- **C**ontext
- **O**utcome
- **T**ime (not always included)

SPICE (Cooke et al. 2012)
- **S**etting
- **P**opulation
- **I**ntervention
- **C**ontrol
- **E**valuation

SPIDER (Cooke et al. 2012)
- **S**ample
- **P**henomena of **I**nterest
- **D**esign
- **E**valuation
- **R**esearch

Cooke et al. 2012 and Methley et al. (2014) reviewed the effectiveness of the extent to which PICO, SPICE and SPIDER are both specific and sensitive in identifying appropriate literature for a qualitative evidence synthesis. Cooke et al. (2012) found that PICO provided the most comprehensive range of results when the key terms and synonyms were combined in a database search. They found that use of SPIDER led to a specific but less comprehensive range of results which could be useful for purposive or selective searching but less useful when exhaustive or comprehensive searching was required. Methley et al. (2014) compared

PICO, SPICE and SPIDER and also concluded that the use of PICO provided the most comprehensive range of results, while SPICE and SPIDER led to a selection of literature. Evaluation of these tools is ongoing. It is unlikely that there will be one tool that is best for all literature reviews, and certainly no tool that will guarantee that you will get all the literature that is relevant to your review question. You are advised to identify the tool whose terms feel the 'best fit' to your study. The most important thing is that the tool enables you to identify a comprehensive range of key terms and synonyms (Tables 4.3 and 4.4). You might find that a combination of the concepts identified in the tools will facilitate this.

Table 4.3 Identifying key terms and synonyms using PICO (quantitative version). Literature review question: Is morphine effective in reducing pain in end-of-life care?

	Population	Intervention	Control	Outcome
PICO term	Palliative care	Morphine	Non-opioids	Reduced pain on pain scale
Alternative terms (synonyms)	Terminal End of life Supportive	Oramorph Narcotic Heroin	Paracetamol NSAID Ibuprofen	Patient comfort Assessment Pain rating scale

Table 4.4 Identifying key terms and synonyms using PICO (qualitative version). Literature review question: Are relatives consulted about pain relief in end-of-life care situations?

	Population	Issue	Context	Outcome
PICO term	Relatives	Pain relief	End-of-life care settings	Experience
Alternative terms (synonyms)	Family Caregivers Carers Next of kin	Analgesia Narcotics	Hospice Palliative care units Terminal care	Feelings Thoughts Perceptions

Electronic database searching

Once you have identified your key terms and synonyms, the next step is to plan your electronic database search. The main approach for all searches is likely to be via electronic databases. There are a vast number of databases which will give you access to a range of different journals. A thorough investigation of available databases will enable you to access the most appropriate for your review. Some databases are specific to the academic discipline in which you work. Some are also freely available without a subscription.

Most academic and hospital libraries will provide a list of databases they subscribe to, together with a description of their content. The names of databases are usually accompanied by a description of each so that you can assess whether it is likely to be relevant to your work. As the availability of databases and their content change on a frequent basis, you are advised to go directly to your academic or hospital library to identify which databases might be appropriate for your search.

Commonly used databases include:

- MEDLINE and PUBMED: extensive medical, nursing and allied health database
- CINAHL: nursing and allied health care with North American and European focus
- EThOS: PhD thesis database
- ZETOC, Open Grey, NHS evidence: databases of grey literature
- PsychINFO: psychology, psychiatry and child development
- Web of Science: includes science citation index and social science citation index

It is advisable to identify as many relevant databases as you can which might hold references relevant to your literature review. This will maximize your chances of identifying appropriate and relevant research and other evidence for your review. We strongly recommend that you avoid use of Google or Google Scholar. This is because these search engines have access to a huge amount of literature that will not be relevant to you and have limited access to academic resources, and hence you are likely to be inundated with many irrelevant hits while not accessing those which are relevant. Restricting your search to Google and Google Scholar will restrict your attempt to identify all the relevant research and other evidence on your topic. We therefore recommend that you limit your use of Google or Google Scholar to the undertaking of a few tasks. Google Scholar can be useful for initial searches in order to assist you with the identification of key terms as well as useful for citation searching, which we discuss later. Google or Google Scholar can also be useful to retrieve full text copies of papers that you have located through more comprehensive database searches, but for which the full copy of the paper is not otherwise accessible. Note that it is often possible to request a full copy from another library, but there is likely to be a cost for this service. Therefore, before you request this, it is always worth a quick Google search to see if the paper is available.

Basics of database searching

It is important that you develop the skills of database searching. This is a complex process and needs practice to refine and time to consider how you might formulate the best search strategies. The aim of database searching is that you identify references to research and other evidence that may be relevant to your literature review question. These references are often referred to as 'hits'.

Ideally your searching on electronic databases will be sensitive enough that you do not identify a large number of irrelevant references and specific enough that you identify papers (hits) that are appropriate for your review.

- If your search is too specific and too sensitive, you will sense that you have only seen the 'tip of the iceberg' and that there are many unlocated hits that might be relevant for your review.
- If your search is not sufficiently specific or sensitive, you will be inundated with references (hits) that are not relevant for your review.

Clearly you are aiming for a middle road that enables you to identify appropriate references from a wider list that is not too extensive. The achievement of this requires a certain amount of skill in searching.

There are two approaches to database searching. The first is using the key terms and synonyms you have identified in a 'free text' search, using the search boxes in the databases. This type of search enables you to use all the key terms you have identified and to be creative about adding new terms to the search as and when they appear, if this fits with your search protocol. You can also choose to search for your key term in the title, abstract or full text, giving you flexibility over the search process. For example, if you are searching for a term which is likely to be given only a brief mention in a paper, then a full text search will pick this up, whereas a search in which the key term was limited to the title or abstract would not. Equally, limiting your search to those papers in which the key term appears in the title or abstract is a useful strategy where you are fairly confident that the key term and the focus of the paper are likely to be similar.

Atkins et al. (2008) illustrate the balance required between getting too many and not enough hits. They describe how, in their study, limiting their search to terms such as adherence and compliance would have focussed the search too much, which might have resulted in the exclusion of studies that might have been relevant. Yet broadening the search would inevitably mean that researchers would have been overwhelmed with results. They acknowledge this as a limitation of their search strategy.

The second approach is to undertake a 'controlled search' using subject headings which have been pre-identified on the database you use. These can be referred to as MeSH or subject headings, but other terms might be used, depending on which database you are using. A controlled search uses subject headings as key terms which have been identified by those compiling the database in order to facilitate the indexing of papers. If you use a controlled search, you will identify papers with key terms that correspond to the pre-identified term. Searching in this way is likely to enable you to locate specific literature but also to lead you to fewer papers, as indexing is limited by the perspective of the professional indexers who are entering papers into the database. The search will also be limited to published papers where the key term is already identified as significant in the paper. Papers which have a simple 'free text' reference to the key term will not be identified using the subject headings as search term and this can significantly affect your search, especially if your key terms are often only a minor focus of a paper but of significant interest to you! Furthermore, searching is often complicated by the imaginative use of clever titles, which can obscure the exact content of papers (Hawker et al. 2002).

Ideally, you should combine both the controlled search and free text search and remove the duplicates that you get. It is advisable to run different searches using different terms and compare the results you get from each one. This will demonstrate that you are taking a thoughtful and reflective approach to your search strategy.

Whichever approach you take, or if you use a combination of both approaches, you need to work out a strategy using the key terms and synonyms you have identified. We discuss how you can do this using the Boolean operators below.

Use of Boolean operators

- AND searches for both terms and hence limits the search.
- OR searches for either term and hence widens the search.
- NOT excludes the term from a search. Many experts recommend caution when using the NOT command in case you omit potentially relevant papers.

The important point here is to beware of using too many ANDs in a search as you might limit your search far too much. It is usually more effective to have a longer list of references and to search through them yourself than to limit your search extensively through use of Boolean operators.

Truncation

Most databases have the * (or equivalent) facility which enables you to place the * at the end of the main stem of the word you are searching for. This will then seek out all the possible endings of the word. A note of caution here though: if you truncate a word too early, for example car* instead of care, you will get many irrelevant hits. Car* is a truncation for car, career, cart, carousel and so on (Table 4.5).

Search limiters

In addition to limiting your search to the key term identification in the title, abstract or full text, there are other limitations you can put on a

Table 4.5 Example of Boolean operators and truncation

Literature review question: What effect does shift length have on the delivery of nursing care?
Nurs* OR Nurse performance OR Nursing care AND Shift pattern* OR Safe staffing OR Rota OR shift

search, including date, language, research type, human or animal, and many others. Careful judgement is needed to assess the relevance of each limiter to your review and it is unwise to restrict your search too far and risk omitting relevant literature. You will find that each database is different, and careful scrutiny of the workings of each is required to find similar limiters in different databases.

Inclusion and exclusion criteria

Most researchers would agree that even with a well-formulated literature review question, clear inclusion and exclusion criteria are useful to guide the identification and selection of literature. Inclusion criteria allow you to specify the remit of your project ,which may not be evidenced in the research question alone. They also provide a clear guide for what you are looking for when you search for literature.

Some inclusion criteria will relate to the type of research and other evidence you need to include. For example, many Cochrane Collaboration reviews of the effectiveness of interventions state that randomized controlled trials will be included and all other research excluded. Other studies might state that only qualitative studies will be included. You need to consider whether country of origin of the study is relevant to your research question: for example, whether there are cultural factors in research that make international studies more or less relevant. You can set limits in most search engines to exclude some of the papers upfront.

Other inclusion criteria will be guided by pragmatic decisions. Date of publication and country of origin of the studies can be a pragmatic approach to limiting the amount of literature included in a study but the limitations of this approach should be acknowledged. There might be important work carried out before the arbitrary cut-off date, or relevant work undertaken in a different country which has been influential to the international and national work undertaken in the area. Pragmatic approaches to defining inclusion and exclusion criteria will be necessary to all levels of post-graduate study but you will need to justify your decisions. If you are going to introduce a cut-off date, it is useful to link it to a key policy change or change in practice, for example the introduction of a new drug.

For example, Candy et al. (2015), in their mixed-methods literature review of the involvement of volunteers in the provision of palliative care services, identified the following inclusion and exclusion criteria for their study.

Inclusion criteria:

- evaluative designs using any comparative method
- non-comparative studies with quantitative analysis such as cross-sectional studies
- qualitative studies that explored the experiences of families
- studies in which participants were terminally ill
- studies which evaluated palliative care services provided by volunteers

Exclusion criteria:

- studies in which patients were chronically ill
- studies which evaluated non-palliative care services
- studies which evaluated the impact of volunteering on the volunteer

An important point to remember is that research and other evidence excluded from your review as a result of the criteria set might be used in different areas of your literature review: for example, in the introduction or discussion. It is not necessarily wasted.

Practice makes perfect

All databases operate slightly differently and it takes time and skill to learn how to use them effectively. You may need a different database strategy for each database. If your library runs training on using databases, make sure you attend as this will assist you to make the most of your searching sessions. You will always pick up new tips even if you are familiar with database searching. The main thing to emphasize with electronic searching is that it is a skill that you need to practise (Just 2012; Smith and Shurtz 2012).

You can test your searching strategies by comparing the results you get using different search terms and different limiters. If a key paper is not identified in one of your searches, you can consider why this is. Doing 'test' searches will help you justify your approach to searching when you write up the method for your literature review. It can be useful to identify five key papers that you would expect your search to identify. If your search does not find them, then this is a good indication that you need to reconsider your search strategy.

Matching your hits with your inclusion criteria

Once you have got a list of hits, or possible relevant research and other evidence from your database searches, you need to match these up with the references which, *prima facie*, seem to fit your inclusion and exclusion criteria. This is an initial match only and we will consider this in a lot more detail in the next chapter.

Assistance from a second reviewer

At this stage, it is useful to engage the assistance of a second reviewer, who you can ask to undertake the same task of comparing the list of results/hits with your inclusion criteria. You can then compare your findings. You can send your second reviewer a copy of your inclusion and exclusion criteria and a copy of your results/hits. Databases often have the facility to share searches between researchers. Your second reviewer can then compare the list of results/hits with the inclusion criteria. You can then assess the level of agreement between you as to the initial inclusion of studies in your review. The second reviewer can be your supervisor, a fellow student or another academic member of staff.

How many hits are too many?

This is a frequently arising question. Ideally, a focussed search should filter out most irrelevant hits but it remains a judgement call regarding how many titles and abstracts you can review from a database. In principle it is wise to err on the side of reviewing a larger number of hits rather than risk overlooking or omitting relevant papers. The process of identifying relevant papers from titles and abstracts can be a quicker process than you might imagine. It is possible to work through many hundred hits in a few hours. So considering the time spent on your project as a whole, and that searching for relevant literature is fundamental to this process, time spent on this activity is probably wisely invested.

An important principle to remember when you are searching is that you do not want to artificially limit the number of hits that you get by narrowing your search too much. While a reduced number of hits might seem more manageable, you need to remember that the aim of the search is to direct you to a comprehensive range of literature, and you need a comprehensive search strategy to facilitate this. If you are truly inundated with hits, for example more than a few thousand, you might consider if the focus of your research question is too broad and whether there is a way that you could limit the focus of the question, while retaining the appropriate depth of literature.

Recording your search results

You need to document the process of refining down your search so that the reader of your work is satisfied that relevant papers have not been omitted on the way. The PRISMA (preferred reporting items for systematic reviews and meta-analyses) flow chart (Figure 4.1) has been developed to help authors of systematic reviews to report their studies in a complete and transparent way, demonstrating the number of references identified and their relevance to the research question (www.prisma-statement.org/statement.htm). There is also a PRISMA checklist, which helps you to report systematic reviews.

If you are submitting your literature review as a requirement for a post-graduate award, those assessing your work may spot-check your searches, taking into consideration that database entries change frequently and databases may merge. Despite this, it should be possible for an external reader of your work to replicate the searches that you have documented.

Common pitfalls in the searching process

Those new to searching often make the following errors when conducting their searches:

1. Using terms that are too specific or too general. You will either get far too few or far too many hits. **For example**, in psychology, the term 'coping' is used so widely you are likely to get directed to an unmanageable amount of hits.
2. Use of too many ANDs. Remember that AND will combine the terms you use and only identify papers which contain both terms. Therefore, if you select a search term that is very focussed and combine this with AND, you are likely to get a very narrow section of hits. The point to remember that not all the words in your literature review question need to be included in your search terms. **For example,** for the literature review question to investigate the impact of intentional rounding on patient safety, key terms would probably be **intentional rounding** and **safety** but would probably not include the term 'impact'. The term 'impact' would limit the search to papers that include this term and there may be relevant papers that do not mention impact specifically.

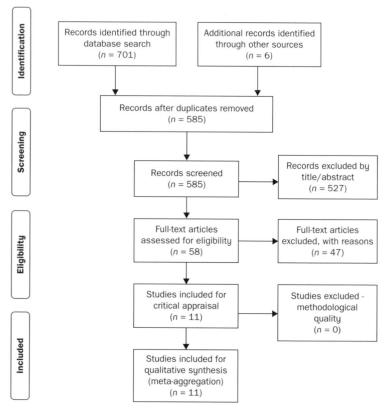

Figure 4.1 An example of a PRISMA diagram, taken from Jakimowicz et al. (2015, p. 26).

3. Inappropriate combinations of words (synonyms) using OR. Remember that all the terms you combine with OR must be representative of the same word. Your search will not work if you combine unassociated words together. **For example**, for the literature review question mentioned above, the following combinations might be made: intentional rounding OR ward round OR handover OR safety. Including safety in the same string of synonyms will make your search less effective.

4. Not enough identified and included synonyms. It is not really possible to have too many OR synonyms. Lots of ORs means that you have thought long and hard about possible synonyms and if they do not

yield any hits, it won't affect your search. **For example**, if you limit your list of synonyms to a few popular terms, you might miss out on papers which have used an alternative term to index the paper.

5. Inappropriate key terms, or failure to state whether key terms are searched for in the title, abstract or whole text. If your key terms are very popular, searching in the whole text will refer you to papers which only give a passing mention to the key terms and you may therefore get a lot of inappropriate papers which do not focus on the topic you are researching. **For example**, it could be good practice to undertake a search using the key terms in the whole text and then compare the hits you get when you restrict the search to the key terms in the title or abstract. Discuss this when you write up your search.

6. Inappropriate use of the truncation * command. This command allows you to search for the stem of a word so that you access all the words that begin with that stem. You need to think carefully about where the truncation command should be placed. **For example**, the words social worker, cannot be truncated down to 'social*' as you will simply get far too many hits.

7. Inappropriate restriction of date and country of publication. Remember that your search should reflect your question and, as such, the restrictions you set on the search must be appropriate to the question. **For example**, there might be important work that has been carried out prior to the dates you set and you need to be mindful of missing significant articles that may be a little older.

Limitations of an electronic search

Most experts agree that using carefully developed key terms will maximize the success of your search strategy (Wong et al. 2004; McKibbon et al. 2006; Wilczynski et al. 2007; Papaioannou et al. 2010). However, there is also agreement that electronic database searching is only the start of your overall literature searching strategy (Wong et al. 2004; Wilcynski et al. 2007; Booth 2008; Langenhoff and Schoones 2011). Due to the limitations of database searching, any search undertaken will not be 100 per cent effective, and a thorough search strategy requires more than a simple electronic search. This conclusion has been reached by researchers who have cross-referenced the results of electronic searching with literature identified in other ways and found that relevant pieces of research were not identified in the results of electronic searches. For example, Betrán et al. (2005) found that only 80 per cent of studies in their review were identified through a database search, and

Mattioli et al. (2012) concluded that although good search terms made the database search more accurate, supplementary searching methods identified more literature. Developing your search to incorporate additional searching techniques will distinguish your search strategy and give your readers confidence that you have accessed a broad range of literature. This is particularly the case for topics which are difficult to search for and where your key terms are not included in the title and abstract of a paper. It is also important where your topic crosses different disciplinary areas and includes policies.

Additional search strategies

The following additional search strategies have been identified and can be considered as supplementary to your electronic database searches.

Additional searching strategies are not 'haphazard' if they are combined with an electronic search. Using these strategies only would be haphazard if they were the *only* means of searching for literature.

Berry picking

Berry picking is an approach to literature searching referred to by Bates (1989), Barroso et al. (2003), and Finfgeld-Connett and Johnson (2013) as part of an expansive literature search, although it could be argued that the approach can be used to enhance any literature search strategy. Berry picking is an ever-changing search for literature in which the researcher 'meanders through the bushes, looking for clumps of berries . . . the searcher wanders through the forest, changing directions as needed to follow up on various leads and shifts in thinking' (Bates 1989). Thus berry picking cannot be described as a linear approach but a process that cannot always be well mapped and which has many twists and turns along the way. The advantage of this approach is that the berry picker (or literature reviewer) can seek out good sources of 'berries' and then search around similar areas where good sources of berries have been found. Peoples et al. (2011) argue that it is not always possible to accurately define and recall the search process and that often one paper will lead to a cluster of useful papers and that the process of achieving this may be difficult to capture. The search strategy cannot always be mapped out from the outset and the way concepts are identified may defy simple reporting. Researchers may also find it hard to remember which route was actually taken.

Citation tracking

If you look up a paper in certain search engines, you can see who else has cited the paper. Useful tools for this are Web of Science or Google Scholar. On Google Scholar, in the bottom right-hand section, you will see a link to cited papers. These papers may be relevant to your review and so a quick assessment of the titles will help you to identify additional papers. This means that you are also less likely to miss the more recent papers.

Searching the reference lists of included papers

Searching the reference lists of papers already identified is a commonly undertaken approach to identifying papers that might have been missed through an electronic search. When you find papers this way, it is useful to track back and see why they were missed by your electronic search. This might give you further ideas about relevant search terms you may have missed.

Hand-searching relevant journals

Hand-searching the contents page of relevant journals is another commonly undertaken approach to identifying papers that might have been missed through an electronic search. You can search either the contents pages, or the complete journal page by page. Again, you might track back and consider why any papers that you find this way were not identified in your electronic search. You can then amend your search strategy to include key terms that have been identified which were not apparent previously.

Author searching

You are likely to find some key authors and researchers who have published in your area. Thus an additional search can be done using the electronic databases in which you search under the authors' name rather than using key terms. This way, you may identify additional research or other evidence published by researchers in the area.

Using automatic targeting systems

Citrome et al. (2009) discuss services which alert you to relevant articles and send you the articles direct to electronic communication.

Lots of journals and databases have 'alerts' lists. For example, the NCBI (National Centre for Biotechnology Information) has a customized profile in which you store key terms. These are searched for you on a regular basis. Really simple syndication (RSS) feeds provide automatic feeds of relevant information. You can also formulate a question and put it online and the papers are directed to you (Citrome et al. 2011).

Locating unpublished literature, including theses and dissertations, monographs, reports, conference abstracts

Depending on the scope of your literature review, these additional search strategies are useful for identifying unpublished material that might lead you onto other significant sources. In addition, contacting the authors of papers that are highly cited in your topic area might lead you to further sources of useful research or other evidence (Flemming et al. 2013).

Books and book chapters

Books and chapters of books are most likely to be useful for background reading for your project but may also be a rich source for the presentation and discussion of theories and concepts that may be related to your work.

Cessation of searching

In any approach to literature searching, it is never completely possible to know when to stop searching. In some approaches, for example for Cochrane Collaboration literature reviews, searching ends once the searching protocol has been completed. For other reviews, cessation of searching is a judgement call as it is never possible to know with any certainty whether all the literature has been located or whether further literature could be found which would contribute significantly to the review and has been missed by a premature end to the searching (Barroso et al. 2003; Booth 2010). However, the approach that you take to the review will provide you with a rationale to end the search. For a comprehensive search, the searching typically ends when all the planned searches have been carried out. For those doing a purposive or selective search, searching typically ends when no new themes are identified in the literature. There might also be limitations due to the scale of the project: for example, due to time or other resources available.

Practicalities for conducting a thorough search

Consider the use of software (for example, Endnote) in which you can save references, abstracts and PDFs. There are also versions which allow you to share references. You can import findings from your searches straight into these reference management systems, although we would recommend limiting your imports to potentially relevant papers to prevent overloading the system. Even citation tracking searches can be entered simply if you set up Google Scholar to allow for 'one click' importing into your reference management system. There are many other alternatives which can be shared. Your learning technologist at your academic institution or your academic librarian will be able to advise you on different options.

Searching for related research and other evidence if there is minimal literature

If your search remains somewhat limited and you do not have sufficient research or other evidence to address your question, you can consider searching for literature that addresses a parallel area. The specific focus you are addressing might not have been researched in your area but might have been explored in relation to a related area: for example, with another population or client group, with a different condition or situation, and so on. It is then possible to draw parallels from the identified literature to address your own literature review question.

In summary

The literature you include in your review is determined by your review question. This is guided by your inclusion and exclusion criteria. Unless you have a good reason not to, we recommend that you undertake a comprehensive search for research and other evidence that meets your inclusion and exclusion criteria. You need to consider that you may have more than one review question and that each will need separate inclusion and exclusion criteria and hence a separate search. A more selective search might be appropriate for additional searches for theoretical or methodological aspects of your review, depending on the findings of your main search.

Searching is a time-consuming process and you need to adopt a clear strategy that will direct you to the appropriate research and other evidence that you can consider for inclusion in your review. This strategy will include searching subject-specific electronic databases in addition to supplementary strategies such as hand-searching journals, author searching, citation searching and wider searches. If you get too many hits, do not artificially reduce them by limiting your search inappropriately, but you may need to reconsider the focus of your search. It is important that you document your search so that others could replicate it if required and that it demonstrates rigour in your study. There is a lot of software that enables you to search, share and store your references. You may be asked to account for your search strategy in an oral examination.

Key points

- You need to undertake a comprehensive search for each question you have identified in your review.
- You may supplement this search with additional searching in order to develop your understanding of theories and methods that may be relevant to your project.
- You need to be able to justify which aspects of your search need to be fully comprehensive and when a more selective search is appropriate.
- Decide on a strategy for your searching, including electronic database searching and additional methods.
- Reconsider your searching approach if you get too many or too few hits.
- Consider software that enables you to search, share results and store your data.
- Ensure this strategy is fully documented within your review.

5

Selection of relevant papers and data extraction

In this chapter we will discuss

- *how you can identify relevant papers for your review*
- *how you can extract and summarize the data which is relevant to your review*
- *how data extraction forms assist with this process*
- *how data extraction forms can be adapted for your individual project*

At this stage, you have completed appropriate searches for your literature review as discussed in Chapter 4, and you should have identified papers that are potentially for inclusion in your literature review. This will usually include empirical research in addition to the relevant discussion of theoretical perspectives and methodological issues where appropriate. The next step is to identify what is relevant for inclusion in your review. In order to make your review as systematic as possible, there are approaches you can follow to ensure rigour in this process. This will prevent your review from becoming an 'ad hoc' collection of studies to one that is clearly and logically thought through and defendable in the written report or oral examination.

This chapter relates most closely to your empirical review, for which you have a clear research question and inclusion and exclusion criteria to guide you. This can be either for a standalone review or one which is a pre-requisite for a larger empirical study. Where you have done additional searches for theoretical and methodological papers to enhance your discussion of theories and methods you have used, your use of data extraction methods may be less extensive.

Selection of possible papers from titles and abstracts

The first step in the selection of papers is to read through the titles and identify those which *prima facie* meet your inclusion criteria, which we discussed in Chapter 4.

You might find that the results of some studies are reported in different papers. Sometimes different aspects of studies are reported in different papers. This can be referred to as 'salami slicing', where researchers understandably seek to maximize the number of possible publications from a study. This practice can also be complicated when researchers in a team rotate authorship of papers which refer to different aspects of their study. A little 'detective work' can usually enable you to determine whether the study described in a paper is the same as that referred to in another paper: for example, if the sample size and location of the study are the same in different papers, this might indicate that the authors are reporting one study in different papers. If it is still unclear, it is possible to contact the authors directly to check. Another potential area for confusion is studies which are initially published as pilot studies and then subsequently published in full. Usually, only the fully documented study will be useful for your literature review although if the pilot study is published in its own right, rather than incorporated into a later study, then it may be eligible for inclusion in the review.

The importance of documenting your method should be flagged up again here. As with all sections of a literature review, it is useful to document what you have done at all stages. This helps to keep the review transparent and rigorous but, more importantly, it keeps a record of what you have done so that you do not repeat tasks unnecessarily, in what can be a complicated process.

It is useful to start to document the process of selection of papers using a flow chart as illustrated in Chapter 4. This will include information about how many hits you had from all of the searches, and how you reduced this number by scanning the titles of each paper. It is also important to document how many duplicate references to the same paper you found on different databases. We have discussed how it is useful to ask a second person to assist you in this task.

Reviewing the titles of each paper alone might not be sufficient to enable you to decide about its relevance to your project and you may want to check the abstract too. This can be done as either a 'one-stage' or 'two-stage' process. You may decide to look at abstracts of potential papers as you find the titles or you may prefer to check titles first and then check the abstracts in a separate check. Not all the databases you use will give you access to an abstract and you may have to access the full paper to get it. Whichever approach you decide to take, it is important to keep a record of abstracts that you have and have not seen, as it is easy to lose track.

Access to the full text of the paper: hard copy or e-copy

Once you have identified the relevant papers from the titles and abstracts, these need further clarification as to whether they fully meet the inclusion criteria you have identified and hence whether or not they should be included in your literature review.

In order to do this, you now need to obtain the full text version or e-copy of the full paper so that further consideration of the relevance and the quality of the paper can be made. If you have not been able to check the abstract, your initial check will be to review the abstract in the first instance, to see if the paper is relevant.

Getting to know your papers

Once you have undertaken an initial check of the full paper, read each paper thoroughly. This might sound like an obvious statement, but understanding the paper is a key point in determining relevance and there are no shortcuts. It is the literature reviewer's equivalent to the qualitative researcher 'getting immersed in the data'. It is not possible to analyse your research and other evidence without a thorough knowledge of the paper. This includes a knowledge of the research design of the papers you are using. As you read the paper, you may find that the research design is not the exact one you are interested in for your review. For example, you might be looking for randomized controlled trials only and the research design you have is quasi-experimental. You might find that the intervention compared in the paper you have is different from the intervention in another paper and you will need to make a judgement as to its relevance to your review. For example, if you are reviewing the effectiveness of music therapy in relieving the symptoms of depression in people with dementia, you will need to consider whether music therapy encompasses the participation in music-making in addition to listening to music. Alternatively, you might find that the population is not relevant for your review. The populations included within a paper might be diverse, or several similar populations may be included within one study. If you are only interested in one sub-population, you will need to consider whether you can access data about the population you are interested in without 'contaminating' your data with information from a population that you are not interested in. These are judgements that you need to make.

Determining the relevance of the paper to your literature review

Once you have got to know your papers well, the next step is to consider the relevance of the paper to your review. We suggest that you do this thoroughly in the first instance so that only papers that are considered relevant are then further critically appraised.

Screening the full paper against your inclusion and exclusion criteria

The first step in identifying relevant papers is to consider the full version of the paper against your inclusion and exclusion criteria. You have already done this with the title and abstract but you now need to consider the paper in full. It is useful to keep a record of this so that you can refer back to this when you write up your method of searching and identification of literature.

A simple inclusion/exclusion criteria tool to facilitate identifying relevant papers can be useful and is shown in Table 5.1. If you use a form such as this you can demonstrate that you have followed a process for assessing whether the paper is relevant to your review.

Table 5.1 Example of a checklist for checking your paper against inclusion and exclusion criteria

---

Inclusion criteria – specifically designed for your review (answers to all questions should be yes)

Example criteria:
- Is the study population over 16 years old?
- Does the study population have symptomatic pleural effusion from an underlying malignant process?
- Does the study compare drug treatments for pleural effusion via the intra-pleural route?
- Is the trial an RCT or a randomized crossover trial?

Exclusion criteria – specifically designed for your review (answers to all questions should be no)

- Does the study include patients with both malignant and non-malignant disease with no clear distinction between the groups in the results?
- Is the study evaluating the effect of a drug administered via a method other than the intra-pleural route?
- Does the study include effusions in a number of different body cavities (for example, peritoneum, pericardium), with no distinction between the groups in the results section?

At this stage the focus of the paper is the key reason for inclusion and a more detailed examination of the papers would follow on those which are included. When you use a summary sheet to assess papers for inclusion and exclusion, a paper trail is created to which you can return rather than going through each paper again.

On this section of the screening form, you are likely to include the following information:

- identification of paper, author(s) and year of publication
- name of person completing the data extraction if part of a larger study
- date of data extraction
- inclusion and exclusion criteria for your literature review

It should be emphasized that these inclusion and exclusion criteria are those developed by you for your own review. It can be useful to add a table and a check box to say whether the paper has met your inclusion and exclusion criteria.

Assistance from a second reviewer

The decision to include or exclude might still not be easy to make and it can be useful to include assistance from a second reviewer at this point. This time, you can ask them to help you identify relevant papers from the full paper, rather than just the title or abstract. This is a useful process in its own right but can be especially useful if you are unsure about the inclusion of a paper; any uncertainty can be settled by consensus with a second reviewer.

Example of a checklist for inclusion and exclusion criteria

In the example given in Table 5.1, the inclusion and exclusion criteria are for a literature review which was conducted as part of a PhD study to explore the effectiveness of treatment in the management of patients with a pleural effusion due to an underlying malignancy. Malignant pleural effusions are the collection of fluid in the pleural space around the lung in a person with a malignancy. It is important to emphasize that these charts must be developed for each individual review and you should be able to defend your rationale for the inclusion and exclusion criteria you set. On the checklist that you create, remember to include a way to identify the study, the authors' names, name of reviewer, date and decision.

For this literature review of the effectiveness of interventions for the reduction of pleural effusion due to malignant disease, the focus is on effectiveness and therefore any studies which do not compare one treatment option against another or a placebo are excluded, even if they are related to the management of pleural effusion and identified in a search. Therefore, only randomized controlled studies which considered the effectiveness of treatment for pleural effusion were included. This was stated in the inclusion criteria for the study. It should be noted that it is not always possible to identify the type of study that will be included in the review. This will depend on the question but requires consideration when you write your inclusion and exclusion criteria and will be reviewed when you write your data extraction form.

Once you have reviewed and selected your papers against your inclusion and exclusion criteria, you will have an almost complete list of papers for inclusion in your review. You can now undertake a detailed assessment of the paper.

This assessment process comprises consideration of two main concepts:

- data extraction
- quality of the paper (critical appraisal)

We will consider data extraction in the remainder of this chapter, and critical appraisal will be discussed in Chapter 6.

Data extraction (data summary)

Data extraction is a process which enables you to extract the relevant information from the papers that are included in your study in preparation for subsequent analysis. Without a logical data extraction process, you will be faced with the task of trying to make sense of the paper without having identified the relevant aspects for your analysis. Pulling out of the individual paper exactly what is relevant to your review will help you prepare your papers for the subsequent process of data analysis.

Data extraction form (data summary form)

A data extraction form (or data summary sheet) is a tool that helps you to manage and process your data (the literature), which will help you select the papers you use for your review and ultimately will help you to write up your literature review. A data extraction (or data summary) sheet can be a useful tool to help you to summarize the key points about a paper and, if this is completed thoroughly, can help you to identify key aspects of the paper that are relevant to your research question and save you from re-reading through each paper every time you want to check on a detail of a paper.

In the data extraction form, you can collect key data from the papers which will help you in three ways:

- to confirm that the paper is relevant for your review
- to focus your thoughts and ideas about the paper
- to provide a summary document about the paper

As with the initial checklist used to identify papers according to the inclusion and exclusion criteria, we suggest that you develop a data extraction sheet that is specific to the needs of your review.

How you use the data extraction sheet will be dependent on your study and you will develop a data extraction sheet that is appropriate for your individual study. Usually it is possible to adapt a data extraction sheet from another project rather than creating your own from scratch. However, your data extraction form will be unique to your individual literature review. There are common features of the form which are likely to be relevant to all studies. An example of a completed data extraction tool is in the appendix.

When you construct your data extraction sheet, you need to make sure that you focus on what is important for your study, otherwise the data extraction will not be 'fit for purpose' and you will find that you keep returning to the original papers. However, it should be pointed out that for some in-depth qualitative studies it might not be possible to capture the main aspects of the study at first read and you might find that you return to the original paper many times before you are confident that you have summarized it appropriately on the data extraction sheet.

The detail with which you undertake this stage will depend on the role of the literature review within your project and the scale of your project. If your literature review is a pre-requisite to an empirical study at MSc level, you will have less scope to develop this aspect of your review than if it is a standalone review or a pre-requisite to an empirical study at PhD level.

You may complete a data extraction sheet for any potential paper that you have identified. There is a note of caution here, however, as you may have a large number of 'possible' papers and it may not be feasible to undertake a full data extraction sheet for each potential paper. You will not know at this stage which papers will be in your final literature review.

We have provided examples of two data extraction forms together with some of the principles that were used to develop the form. The first example (Table 5.2) is a quantitative form and the second example (Table 5.3) is a qualitative form. We have provided a completed data extraction form in the appendix.

Example of a data extraction form for a systematic review of randomized controlled trials (RCTs)

You can see from the example of the data extraction form that a carefully constructed form will enable you to pull out very detailed information

Table 5.2 Data extraction form for a systematic review of randomized controlled trials

Details about the study			
Country or countries			
Start of recruitment			
End of recruitment			
Intended duration of follow-up for each patient (months) – please state maximum			
Number of recruiting centres			
If >1 recruiting centres, is the trial cluster randomized? (Yes/No/NA)			
Type of report (F = full text; A = abstract; U = unpublished)			
Language			
What is the study evaluating? (A = pleurodesis agent; B = mode of admin of pleurodesis; C = other method to optimize pleurodesis; D = IPC)			
Details of the intervention			
Common treatment for all groups (therefore not under comparison)			
Group	**1**	**2**	**3**
Description of intervention			
Dose			
Number of doses given and frequency			
Mode of administration			
Number of patients randomized			
Number lost to follow-up and reasons			
Which group was used as the control? (tick one)			
How did you decide which was the control group? (tick one)	Assumed by data extractor ☐		
	Stated in paper ☐		

Table 5.3 Data extraction form for a qualitative or mixed-method systematic review

Author (year), country, score	Research question or aim of study	Details about the study			Key themes
		Participants	Method	Palliative care team	
Dharmasena and Forbes (2001), UK, 25	Will doctors refer non-cancer patients to palliative care?	78 consultants	Postal survey, 8 items. Analysis not described.	Not described	Model of care; professional onus; expertise and trust; skill building vs. deskilling
Salomon et al. (2001), France, 30	To describe the current management of terminally ill patients from care providers' viewpoint	31 physicians, 16 nurses	Structured, self-administered, 33-item survey. SPSS (statistical package for the social sciences) used for analysis	Physician, nurse, psychologist	Model of care; skill building vs. deskilling; specialist palliative care operations
Carter et al. (2002), New Zealand, 29	To determine health professionals' perception of the service's impact on patients, families and staff, and areas that need improvement	127 doctors, 242 nurses, 11 social workers	Postal survey, 5-point Likert scale and yes/ no questions. EPI6 used for analysis.	Full-time nurse, part-time physician	Model of care; skill building vs. deskilling; specialist palliative care operations

about the study. It is not possible to know in advance which data you have extracted you will use in your final analysis; some papers might have minimal reference to the details you are interested in and you will not know this until you have gone through all the papers. Therefore, you will extract more data than you eventually use in your analysis. Once you have established the type(s) of study design (if appropriate), you need to identify which details about the study design you need to report. For this study, the researchers required information about trial design: for example, whether design was a cluster design or a simple random-ized controlled design. In addition, they required information about the intervention; with a drug trial, this is about drug dose and frequency, but with another form of intervention, such as a service-delivery model, the intervention needs to be clearly documented. You also need to consider how the success, or not, of the intervention was defined and measured. It is not always clearly stated in a paper how an outcome has been mea-sured, and you might consider contacting the authors of the paper if this is not identified. In this literature review, the primary outcome could be described as the complete removal of fluid, as identified on x-ray or by the absence of symptomatic signs of fluid. Some papers, especially those published longer ago, might not record any detailed information in this and merely report a successful drainage of fluid without an accom-panying definition. Much of this information needs to be assessed and clarification sought from the authors if possible. The primary outcome measure from your review may be different from the primary outcome of the paper as it may be a secondary outcome measure. You will have decided upon your primary outcome for the review but also some secondary outcome measures and adverse event reporting.

If you are going to do a meta-analysis, decisions have to be made about what to accept as a 'good enough' result to use in the analysis. Absolute values are then recorded according to the number randomized in each arm, numbers analysed in each arm and those lost to follow up. This is important to assess for bias in the study. For more details on extracting data for RCTs see the *Cochrane Handbook for System-atic Reviews of Interventions* (Higgins and Green 2011). For before and after study designs, and quasi-experimental or controlled studies, similar data will be collected.

Data extraction form for qualitative or mixed-methods studies

Data extraction forms for qualitative and mixed-method studies are slightly different, as the process of analysing literature data tends to be more iterative and less of a 'one-off' event. The way in which you develop your data extraction form for qualitative research papers will depend on the approach you intend to take for the analysis. If there is a large body of work that has already been undertaken in an area, your analysis of the literature can be undertaken deductively. In this case, it is possible to pre-specify themes from the existing body of literature which will be searched for in the different papers that make up your review. Those undertaking a framework analysis, which we discuss in Chapter 7, use this approach. In this case, you can tailor your data extraction form to pre-specify the areas of interest you are searching for. More usually, however, data analysis is inductive, where the reviewers retain an open stance to the literature and identify themes as they arise from the papers rather than imposing a pre-established framework. In this case, it is not possible to pre-state concepts in a data extraction sheet, as you will not be aware what these concepts will be until you have read the research. However, you can develop this form so that you can create a table to which you can extract the themes arising in your data straight away. Remember tables can be used to describe your data and highlight themes but the craft of your synthesis will come in how you discuss and synthesize the findings from the tables. We will discuss this further in Chapter 7.

As with all research, you need to read and re-read the paper to ensure that you have a thorough understanding of what it is about, and you need to ensure that you stay close to the data at all times. What, at first glance, may seem to be an appropriate interpretation of a paper might be revised on later reading and in comparison with other papers, when your understanding of the research area has developed.

We have provided another example of a data extraction form in Table 5.3 together with some of the principles that were used to develop the form. The purpose of this literature review was to explore the perceptions of services from those who were experiencing a life-limiting illness.

You can see from the example of the qualitative data extraction form in Table 5.3 that, as with the quantitative data extraction form, a carefully constructed form will enable you to pull out very detailed information about the study. In this study, researchers were interested in the perceptions of services of those with a life-limiting condition, and they had used both qualitative and quantitative research to address this question. Because of the broad focus of the research, data extraction had to be selective and relevant to the literature review question.

It is important to find out about who the participants are so that you can understand the context in which the findings or themes are discussed. It is useful to retain as much context as possible to avoid misinterpretation of the data at the analysis stage. It is useful to extract as much of this information as possible.

In this study, methods used to explore users' perception are varied. You need to record the approach taken in the study, including data collection and analysis approaches. The data extraction table needs to be able to accommodate a variety of methods rather than just having tick boxes. This is especially important in qualitative methods, where the approaches used are often diverse and might have been adapted to suit the needs of the study.

You need to identify the key themes that arise in relation to your review question. You might choose to provide these in detail on the data extraction form or you might consider this in another table. Sometimes the key themes that have been identified by the researchers in their analysis of their data will be relevant to your review but this depends on your review question. You might identify alternative themes or re-name the themes used in the paper.

Sample data extraction for non-research evidence

Depending on your inclusion and exclusion criteria, you might find that you have included non-research papers in your review. In this case, you will need to extract data from these in a similar way to what you have done for the research papers included in the review. As with all papers, it is important to extract only the data which are relevant to answering your review question.

You might find it useful to develop a data extraction form for evidence other than research papers that you include in your review (Table 5.4). The same principles apply; the purpose of the data extraction form is to provide clarity and a standardized approach to the evidence you have so that you can use it in your subsequent analysis.

Table 5.4 Data extraction form for non-research

Author (year) country	Type of evidence	Type of arguments	Main outcomes
Who wrote the paper, when and where?	Is the evidence discussion or a more developed theory?	How are the arguments expressed?	What are the main messages?

Pilot testing the data extraction forms

Once you have developed the full data extraction form, you are ready to start in earnest. At this point we suggest that you identify two papers that you are fairly confident are papers that are highly likely to be included in your review. You can use these to model or test out your data extraction form.

The data extraction form will usually revisit the initial inclusion and exclusion criteria. This is because when the paper is examined in more detail, you might find that it is then excluded from your review. It is also possible that some papers might have been rejected inappropriately at the initial data extraction stage, which is why you need to remain open to the possibility of returning to the original papers at any stage of your literature review.

Once you have tested out your data extraction form, we suggest that you and a colleague, or member of the review team if you have one, review up to five papers independently of each other. You can then come together to see if you have completed the forms in similar ways. You may notice that the second reviewer has interpreted some of your data extraction questions in a different way. You may also notice you have missed some vital pieces of information which initially you might not have wanted to collect – such as length of hospital stay, cost or mortality data – which you hadn't been expecting to be recorded. At this point further sections to add clarity can be added to the form.

Following this, you should have a data extraction form that is pilot tested and that you are confident will help you to summarize the data from the literature you intend to include in your review. We suggest that you complete a data extraction form for each study that you have identified as potentially relevant for your review and that you document this when you write up your method.

In summary

Once you have identified which papers meet the inclusion and exclusion criteria that you have set for your review, the next step is to read the papers thoroughly and extract the details of the papers that are relevant for your review. This is usually done with your empirical literature but the process can be useful when you are reviewing theories and concepts in your review. This process is often referred to as data extraction, and the purpose is to organize and standardize the data so that you can see clearly how they relate to your review question. Data extraction is concerned with exploring the detailed results from a study you are intending to include in your literature review. The data extraction process helps you to process the results of the research or other evidence you have and to clarify your understanding of the paper. It is useful to develop a data extraction sheet so that you can summarize the results of the papers onto one form. This serves two purposes: it provides clarity about the papers and it prevents you from having to refer back to the original studies. Data extraction is different from critical appraisal, which we will explore in the next section.

Key points

- Papers you have identified as possible for selection in your review need to be compared against your inclusion and exclusion criteria.
- Papers that meet your inclusion criteria need to be carefully considered to check they are relevant to your review.
- In order to focus on the detail of the included papers, data extraction sheets can be developed.
- Data extraction is a useful way to prepare your papers for subsequent data analysis.
- These need to be specific to the individual study but can be adapted from other studies.
- Data extraction is a separate process from critical appraisal.

6

Critical appraisal of the literature

In this chapter we will discuss:
- *the importance of identifying the strengths and weaknesses of the papers you include*
- *considerations to make when appraising quantitative and qualitative research*
- *different tools that might assist with the process of critical appraisal*
- *the importance of using the critical appraisal when you analyse and synthesize the papers*

Once you have read all of the papers that are relevant for your review and undertaken a data extraction process, where appropriate, the next stage is critical appraisal of the papers.

What is critical appraisal

Critical appraisal is the process of carefully and systematically assessing the quality of the literature, in which you have to judge its trustworthiness and value in a particular context (Burls 2009). It is important to consider how the research has been conducted and the strengths and weaknesses of the other evidence you are considering for inclusion in your review, because you need to make a judgement about the quality of the evidence and hence the weight it should have when you analyse and synthesize the papers. Incorporating poorly designed studies, or to give them the same weight as a stronger study, can be misleading and can affect the results of your review (Tong et al. 2007). Therefore you need to consider how to how to deal with the stronger and weaker studies in your review.

A common error that many students make is that they undertake a critical appraisal of the studies but then do not make use of the critical appraisal in the subsequent analysis and synthesis of literature. Critical appraisal is only useful if you use it in your analysis. We will discuss this in Chapter 7.

The important point to make about critical appraisal is that it is not an end in itself. It is not a standalone component of a review which needs to be done and then promptly dismissed. The purpose of critical appraisal is to be incorporated into your data analysis and synthesis, and you must take into account the impact of both the stronger and weaker studies. This requires a value judgement, which you will need to justify when you consider your analysis and synthesis of your literature (discussed in Chapter 7) and when you write up your literature review (discussed in Chapter 8).

The following example illustrates how critical appraisal of studies that you consider for inclusion in your review can have a significant impact on the results of the review. In this example, omitting studies which had been less well conducted dramatically changed the outcome of the systematic review.

Inclusion and exclusion of studies in a literature review according to quality assessment

In Chapter 1 we referred to the different outcomes of two systematic reviews which were undertaken to analyse the effectiveness of mammography in preventing mortality from breast cancer. The first systematic review (Gøtzsche and Nielsen 2011) surveyed a wide range of studies, including those with weaker methods, that compared the mortality rate of women who had had a mammography for the early detection of breast cancer with those who had not. The researchers came to the conclusion that the benefit of mammography in preventing breast cancer deaths was marginal. Because of the controversy this outcome provoked, a second systematic review was undertaken. In the second review (Marmot et al. 2012) the researchers made different decisions about the inclusion of older, less well-conducted studies and included only those studies which they judged to have used stronger methods. Their review came to a different conclusion.

> By excluding the weaker studies, Marmot et al. (2012) found that those women who underwent mammography breast screening had approximately a 20 per cent lower risk of dying from breast cancer.

The important point is that the inclusion of stronger and weaker studies in your review can have a major impact on the outcome. This illustrates the importance of appraising the strengths and weaknesses in the literature you have and how you will use the stronger and weaker studies in your subsequent analysis and synthesis.

Assessing quality and risk of bias

Given the importance of undertaking a quality assessment in the research and other evidence you include in your review, the next question is how this should be done. While there is agreement that considerations of quality must be made, the question of what constitutes quality is not so easy to resolve. Quality assessment both for qualitative and quantitative research and for other evidence can be a complex process and we discuss this below. It is because of the continuing debate about quality assessment that we advise you to undertake the quality assessment only once you have confirmed that the research or other evidence is relevant for your review and you have completed the data extraction process. In this way, you critically appraise only the papers that you intend to use within your review and do not consider the quality of literature that may not be relevant to your literature review. Quality assessment is then undertaken once you have established that a piece of research or other evidence is relevant to your review.

The process of critical appraisal does not necessarily include the use of a tool, but these can be useful and we will discuss this later in this chapter. The appraisal process is similar regardless of the type of analysis you undertake. Critical appraisal is the process of identifying how well the research has been conducted.

Quality standards in quantitative studies

In quantitative research methods, there has been a long tradition of developing and testing research methods so that we now know the optimum ways of conducting the research. In quantitative research there is homogeneity about fundamental principles such as the nature of truth and reality, and this leads to principles that focus on the risk that many different factors can lead to potential bias in the study. Studies are assessed according to these different areas of potential risk, and an overall assessment of risk of bias can be given as high, unclear or low.

For example, Sibbald and Roland (1998) described the process of undertaking a randomized controlled trial (RCT) and the essential steps involved:

- There is random allocation.
- Participants and clinicians are unaware of treatment allocation if possible.
- Intervention groups are managed in the same way as the control group.
- Participants are analysed in the group they were allocated to.
- Analysis is focussed on estimating the difference in size in pre-determined criteria.

Subsequently there has been much discussion, and some research has been undertaken into determining optimum ways to carry out the randomization process: for example, with the use of a truly random method such as a computer program, or an approach that conceals any randomization list so that the clinical team cannot second guess which allocation the next participant will receive (Schulz and Grimes 2002; Akoberg 2005).

Further information on risk of bias can be found in the Cochrane Collaboration *Handbook* (Higgins and Green 2011). The Cochrane Collaboration has developed a bias assessment tool (Higgins and Green 2011), which focusses on the assessment of the potential sources of bias as identified above.

In questionnaire design, to take another example, there are generally agreed principles regarding rigour in the development and administration of the questionnaire. These are discussed by Leung (2001) in a linked Cochrane resource. The keys areas to consider in a questionnaire study are:

- the design of the questionnaire
- the testing of the questionnaire
- the administration of the questionnaire
- the sample that will complete the questionnaire

When the key features of a research design are established, you can use them as a benchmark against which you can compare the studies you identify and draw a conclusion about the quality of the research you have. For example, you might decide to include only questionnaires which have a particular outcome measure based upon psychometric properties, and those tested more robustly would be included over others or given more weight.

In addition to knowledge and understanding of quantitative research methods, various statements and checklists have also been put in place to standardize approaches to quality. For example the CONSORT statement, which was originally developed as a tool to enhance quality in the publication of RCTs, can also be used as a tool to measure quality of the RCT (Tong et al. 2007). There are also many critical appraisal tools which focus on the assessment of quality of quantitative studies, which we will describe later in this chapter.

Quality standards in qualitative studies

In qualitative research, as in quantitative methods, research and debate about optimal methods are ongoing. However, because there is more heterogeneity in the methods used, agreement about quality is more elusive. The difficulty of using predetermined quality standards for qualitative research and avoiding ritualistic approaches is discussed by many researchers (Cleary et al. 2014). This is because of the wide diversity in qualitative approaches which have been developed as a response to the need to research a varied range of research questions. Qualitative approaches need to be flexible and creative enough to meet the methodological demands of the study. For example, Wiles et al. (2011) identified 57 qualitative studies published between 2000 and 2009 which claimed to have developed innovative approaches in response to the individual needs of the qualitative designs. Shin et al. (2009) also identify a wide range of methods and strategies incorporated into what they described as qualitative research. However, while qualitative research designs need to be flexible, they must also retain academic rigour. Whittemore et al. (2001) argue that 'creativity must be preserved within qualitative research but not at the expense of the quality of the science' (p. 526). Debate exists as to what constitutes reasonable deviation from an established approach in response to study need (Aveyard and Neale 2009). Such diversity leads to the need for a broad range of quality indicators in qualitative research.

Assessment of quality in qualitative research: flexible guidelines and transparency

Lincoln and Guba (1985) argue that qualitative research should be assessed in terms of credibility, transferability, dependability and confirmability, and suggest that these are more appropriate for assessing the quality of a qualitative study than terms such as the more traditional 'validity' and 'reliability', which are used within quantitative research. Lincoln and Guba (1985) argue that all qualitative research should have a 'truth value' and that this could be determined by strategies that represent the hallmark of good qualitative research, such as keeping an accurate trail of the research process and transparency in the data analysis process, rather than specifications about the process of conducting the research *per se*. This seminal work set a precedent for openness and transparency in the reporting of qualitative studies.

Walsh and Downe (2006) also argue that transparency and openness are the quality standards for qualitative research. In their literature review of the way in which quality is assessed in qualitative studies, the authors identified eight existing checklists and frameworks. From their analysis of these checklists and frameworks, they also argue that the assessment of qualitative research should incorporate an identification of a method which is consistent with the intent of the research, researcher reflexivity, ethical dimensions, literature review and an analytical approach.

Spencer et al. (2003) identified four central principles for guiding the assessment of qualitative research. These were:

- contributory to our understanding
- defensible in design
- rigorous in conduct
- transparent and systematic

These principles focus on description and rationale for the approaches followed rather than prescription of approaches, although they do indicate other quality issues such as that interviews should be tape recorded and context of data should be preserved.

Tong et al. (2007) published their *Consolidated Criteria for the Reporting of Qualitative Studies* and emphasized the importance within qualitative research of discussion of the research team and reflexivity, the study design, and analysis and findings.

In their review of the quality assessment of qualitative studies for research into adapted physical activity, Zitomer and Goodwin (2014) identified various approaches to the assessment of quality in 56 papers and argued for a set of 'flexible guidelines' rather than rigid criteria to guide the assessment of qualitative research. They identified the concepts of credibility, resonance, significant contribution, ethics and coherence as relevant to the assessment of qualitative research.

The QARI tool for assessing qualitative studies is published by the Joanna Briggs Institute (2014) and focusses on three elements of qualitative research:

- whether there is congruity between the philosophy, methodology, method, presentation of data and their interpretation
- whether bias and assumptions made are explicit
- whether the relationship between what the participants report to have said and the conclusions of the study is clearly made

These examples illustrate that the assessment of quality in qualitative studies has a clear focus on the transparency of reporting and flexibility of approaches rather than on defining specific rules for the conduct of qualitative research. While this captures the essence of qualitative research it falls short of giving definitive guidance on what the reviewer should be looking for in terms of quality indicators when considering the merits of a qualitative study.

Incorporating qualitative studies in a literature review

While the focus on flexibility and transparency gives much room for the discretion of the researcher in the development of quality in the study, it also gives the same discretion to the reviewer in how to consider the assessment of quality when including qualitative studies in a review. The benchmarks for quality are open to interpretation and it can be difficult for the literature reviewer to decide which studies they should include on the basis of quality. As a result, there is a divide of opinion in the research literature regarding how to judge the quality of qualitative studies and whether or not they should be excluded from a literature review on the basis of quality. One approach is to exclude studies on the basis of a pre-determined quality assessment. Examples of organizations and individuals who follow this approach are the Joanna Briggs Institute (2014), Harden (2007) and Walsh and Downe (2006).

Another approach is to include all studies into the review, irrespective of the perceived quality. Researchers who have followed this approach include Petticrew and Roberts (2005), Bondas and Hall (2007), Dixon-Woods et al. (2007), Noyes and Popay (2007), Atkins et al. (2008),

Thomas and Harden (2008), Finfgeld-Connett (2014), Giles and Hall (2014), Smiddy et al. (2015) and Rock et al. (2015).

Critical appraisal tools for assessing quality

The debates about the assessment of quality of research, especially in relation to qualitative studies, will not be resolved within the times-cale of your post-graduate project, and you need to find a pragmatic approach to incorporating issues of quality. In order to assist with this, many critical appraisal tools have been developed for the assessment of research, and these can be a useful aide to determining the quality of an individual research study. In addition to critical appraisal tools for research, there are also critical appraisal tools for assessing the quality of arguments, theories, and guidelines and policy. They are not an essential requirement of any post-graduate project, however, and do not replace your own careful consideration of the research and other evidence you use.

There are many critical appraisal tools available. Back in 2004, Katrak et al. identified over one hundred critical appraisal tools available in the literature but concluded that many of these lacked a rigorous evaluation of their effectiveness; they argued that the proliferation of appraisal tools had not been accompanied with a thorough assessment of their value. In 2012, Hannes and Macaitis identified 24 different assessment tools that were commonly used in studies. They also found a varying ability among the commonly used critical appraisal tools to trigger the identification of methodological weaknesses of the research reviewed. In view of the many appraisal tools available, you are very likely to find a tool that is directly related to the specific study you need to appraise. This tool might encourage you to think critically about the study.

Some studies have been undertaken that have compared the critical evaluation of studies by researchers both with and without the use of an appraisal tool. For example, Dixon-Woods et al. (2007) compared the use of two checklists and the unprompted judgement of the reader in the conclusions made about a qualitative paper. They did not find that structured appraisal tools yielded more agreement about the quality of the study than unprompted judgement, although those using structured tools were more explicit in their reasons for their judgements.

The conclusion is that critical appraisal tools are not an essential component of the process of critical appraisal and there is no one 'gold standard'. Burls (2009) argues that checklists are useful not as a replacement for thought and judgement but as an 'aide memoire' (p. 3) when considering the strengths and weaknesses of a study design. In view of this, we argue that critical appraisal tools are a useful aid to triggering thought and judgement about a research paper or other evidence. They are not a definitive route to a comprehensive assessment. It is probably beneficial to use a critical appraisal tool but to be aware that there is no one recommended tool and that a critical appraisal tool is not a substitute for a thorough knowledge and understanding of the research or other evidence you are evaluating.

Examples of critical appraisal tools for empirical research

Due to the widespread availability and choice of critical appraisal tools, there are many ways to access them. One of the most useful websites is that provided by the University of South Australia, which gives links to a wide variety of critical appraisal tools for research and other sources of evidence; at time of writing this is available at www.unisa.edu.au/research/sansom-institute-for-health-research/research-at-the-sansom/research-concentrations/allied-health-evidence/resources/cat.

There are critical appraisal tools which are specific to the research designs, for example the Critical Appraisal Skills Programme (CASP) guidelines and those published by the Joanna Briggs Institute (2014), which publishes critical appraisal checklists for a range of studies (qualitative studies are included in one checklist). These checklists are available online at www.casp-uk.net and www.joannabriggs.org.

Other critical appraisal tools are more general, refer to qualitative or quantitative research designs (rather than individual research designs), and are referenced in journal articles or textbooks: for example, Law et al. (1998), Walsh and Downe (2006), Coughlan et al. (2007), Ryan et al. (2007) and Beck (2009). A critical appraisal tool for mixed-method studies has been developed by Hawker et al. (2002), in which they recommend researchers grade the following aspects of a study from good to very poor and comment on their reason for doing so:

- abstract and title
- introduction and aims
- method and data
- sampling
- ethics and bias
- findings/results
- transferability and generalizability
- implications and usefulness

Other critical appraisal tools can be found by a simple Google search or perhaps referred to in other research textbooks and journal articles. Some critical appraisal tools provide a method of scoring a study while others provide a checklist but without a final score. Whichever type of appraisal tool you use, the important thing is that you use it to determine the strength of evidence that your paper provides for your study.

For those undertaking a systematic review with a meta-analysis, the Cochrane Collaboration discourages the use of scales and checklists for assessing quality. While the approach offers an appealing simplicity, it is not supported by empirical evidence (Emerson et al. 1990; Schulz et al. 1995). Calculating a summary score inevitably involves assigning 'weights' to different items in the scale, and it is difficult to justify the weights assigned. Higgins and Green (2011) argue that it is preferable to use simple approaches for assessing validity that can be fully reported. The Cochrane Collaboration has developed a risk of bias assessment tool for use within a systematic review which incorporates RCTs (Higgins and Green 2011). This assessment tool focusses on the assessment of the risk of bias in the following areas: generation of allocation sequence, concealment of allocation, blinding, attrition, generic biases, biases specific to the trial, biases of the clinical speciality.

Examples of critical appraisal approaches for non-research evidence

In addition to critical appraisal tools for empirical research, there are tools for assessing the quality of other evidence such as theories, guidelines, government reports, and discussion or argument papers. Given the influence and importance that some non-research litera-ture can have, it is important that you subject it to as much scrutiny as empirical research (Bradshaw 2015). Therefore when you include non-research evidence in your review, it is important that you assess the quality of it in an appropriate way. For example, Dunleavey (2015, via email) undertook a systematic review to explore the barriers and facilitators to patient and carer recruitment to RCTs in palliative care. The data for this study came only from the results of trials but also from the discussion sections, where the researchers published their reflections on the process of recruitment. Some discussions will be stronger and more logical than others and this can be assessed within a critical framework. Examples of appraisal tools for non-research evi-dence are given below.

Fawcett (2005) proposes criteria for the evaluation of theories and suggests that they can be considered according to:

- significance
- internal consistency
- clarity
- testability
- confirmability with empirical research

Bradshaw (2015) has provided a framework against which government reports can be evaluated and suggests the following criteria, which are based on the framework proposed in Thiselton (2012):

- the value judgements made by the writer of the report
- the accessibility of the report to a lay reader
- consideration of the perceptions of the reader
- the intention to change perceptions
- the reliability of data used in the report
- consideration of historical underpinnings
- the intention of the report

The AGREE Collaboration (at time of writing, located at www.agree-trust.org/about-the-agree-enterprise/agree-research-teams/agree-collaboration) provides assessment criteria for the evaluation of clinical guidelines. The aim of the criteria is to assess the methodological rigour and transparency with which the guidelines have been developed. The criteria have six domains:

- scope and purpose
- stakeholder involvement
- rigour of development
- clarity
- applicability
- editorial independence

Caraceri et al. (2012) provide an example of the review and evaluation of guidelines undertaken by a panel of experts for the European Association of Palliative Care (EAPC) on the use of opioids in the treatment of cancer pain. The experts reviewed the previous EAPC guidelines and compared these against currently available guidelines. Consensus recommendations were reached by an expert panel.

Cottrell (2011) proposes criteria for the evaluation of arguments and discusses how the author's position, line of reasoning and intention to persuade can be used to assess the quality of an argument. This approach builds on the work of Thouless and Thouless (1953), who articulate 38 'dishonest tricks' commonly used in argument, such as:

- using emotionally charged words
- making statements using words such as 'all' when 'some' would be more appropriate
- using selected instances
- misrepresentation of opposing arguments
- evasion of a sound refutation of an argument

How to use the critical appraisal within your literature review

The process of critical appraisal and the use of critical appraisal tools are well established within academic institutions, and many students commencing post-graduate study will be familiar with the concept. It can be tempting to see critical appraisal as an 'end in itself' rather than a method which will assist your ongoing analysis and synthesis of literature. When you undertake your critical appraisal, it is important that you make a judgement about the overall strengths and weaknesses of the research or other evidence that you have so that you can use this judgement in your subsequent analysis and synthesis.

In summary

Critical appraisal enables you to identify the strengths and weaknesses of a paper and hence determine the weight each paper should play in your subsequent analysis. We argue that an appropriate critical appraisal tool can be a useful way of considering quality issues in a research paper. However, it is important to remember that the process of critical appraisal is not synonymous with the use of a tool. The use of a tool should prompt you to think critically about the research or other evidence you are using for your review. You can also think critically about the literature without the use of a tool. Use of a critical appraisal tool does not replace sound knowledge of the research methods used in the paper, without which it is not possible to appraise it. The importance of any tools is largely that they help you to get to know the papers and identify the strengths and weaknesses. There are many critical appraisal tools available; you may find it helpful to use a tool which is specific to the research design you are using rather than a generic tool. In recent years, the Cochrane Collaboration have moved away from the use of traditional critical appraisal tools towards tools which focus explicitly on the risk of bias. Those undertaking a systematic review with meta-analysis are advised to refer to Higgins and Green (2011) risk of bias assessment tool. What is important is that once you have undertaken the critical appraisal of each study, and have identified the strengths and weaknesses of the research study, you need to decide how you will use this appraisal in your literature review. We will discuss this in Chapter 7.

Key points

- Critical appraisal enables you to determine the strengths and weaknesses of the papers in your review.
- Critical appraisal or risk of bias tools can be a useful aid to this process.
- It is possible to appraise a paper without the use of a tool.
- Critical appraisal does not replace the need to understand the methods used in a paper.
- Critical appraisal is not a 'standalone' activity.
- Critical appraisal is only useful if you use it within your subsequent data analysis and synthesis.

7

How do I analyse and synthesize my literature?

In this chapter we will discuss:
- *the different approaches to the analysis and synthesis of literature*
- *how the approach to analysis and synthesis depends on the method you undertake for your review*
- *the approach to meta-analysis*
- *different approaches to qualitative and mixed-method analysis*
- *common features of qualitative and mixed-method analysis of literature*

By this point, you will have selected the research and other evidence that are relevant for your literature review. These will be the research papers and other evidence that meet your inclusion criteria, which may have stated methodological requirements for inclusion in the review. You will have undertaken a data extraction and a critical appraisal of all included studies. You will now have a working knowledge of which are the stronger and weaker papers in your review. You are now ready to analyse and synthesize your literature.

> analysis: breaking down the parts in order to understand the individual components
>
> synthesis: building up the parts into a coherent whole

Data extraction and critical appraisal of your papers are the first stage of analysis. You will continue your analysis when you look closely at the details of what each paper can tell you about your review question. In your synthesis, you will build a picture of what all the papers can tell us about your review question.

Different methods of analysis and synthesis are required for different types of data; that is, whether you have quantitative or qualitative research, or a mixture of both and (or) other evidence. You will be familiar with the data analysis used in quantitative and qualitative research. In quantitative research, data is often analysed and synthesized numerically, using statistical tests, whereas in qualitative research, texts are analysed and synthesized using a narrative approach. The same principles are applied to the analysis and synthesis of literature in a review.

Quantitative papers which are sufficiently similar can be analysed and synthesized using statistical analysis known as a meta-analysis or descriptive statistics. Qualitative and mixed-methods papers can be analysed and synthesized thematically and there are many approaches to doing so. As mentioned in Chapter 2, there are methodological discussions about the appropriateness of combining different qualitative approaches (Atkins et al. 2008), but there is general agreement that the utility of bringing evidence together in an analysis and synthesis outweighs consideration of loss of context, if the review is undertaken rigorously.

Going beyond describing the content of original studies is often referred to as the defining characteristic of analysis and synthesis (Harden et al. 2004). It is the main purpose of a literature review to bring all the results of the studies together in an appropriate analysis and synthesis. The way in which you undertake this analysis and synthesis of your literature depends on the type of literature that you have and the approach to literature review that you have undertaken.

In this chapter, we will discuss the analysis of literature using statistical measures and non-statistical approaches (Figure 7.1).

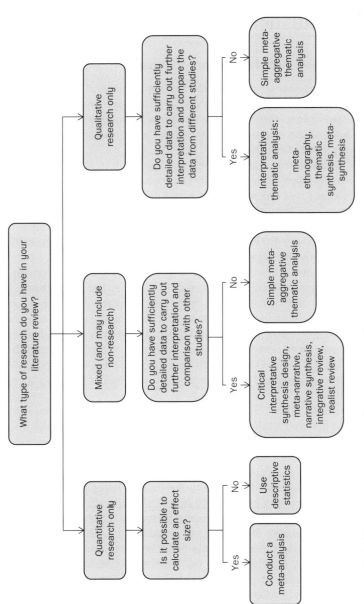

Figure 7.1 Different approaches to the analysis of literature

Approaches to analysis of the literature using statistical measures

Meta-analysis and descriptive analysis

Meta-analysis may be appropriate for your review if the papers you have for analysis adopt a similar method and have similar outcomes. It may be possible to combine these in a meta-analysis. This is a statistical re-analysis of the original statistics in the individual papers to provide one overall statistical result.

In the same way that the Cochrane approach to systematic review was the forerunner of the literature review as a formal research method, meta-analysis was one of the first formal and standardized approaches to data analysis. Meta-analysis is an approach to data analysis which you can use if you have mainly similar quantitative studies (often randomized controlled trials or RCTs) where it is possible to combine the results of all of the studies into one overall result.

Meta-analysis has been very important in the development of evidence-based practice. In the example given earlier in this book, the effectiveness of Streptokinase, a drug used in the treatment of myocardial infarction, was identified through a meta-analysis of many small clinical trials (Mulrow 1994). Due to the small size of each trial, most did not find conclusive results in favour of the use of Streptokinase. However, when the trials were brought together in a meta-analysis, and the results were pooled and re-analysed, the true effect of the drug became apparent.

A meta-analysis relates to how we combine findings from similar studies to get an overall outcome, based on a summary of all the results of all studies. This means that effect sizes of individual studies can be combined to form a summary statistic to show the effect size across studies. Typical effect sizes used are risk ratio, relative risk and odds ratio. This is only possible when studies include outcome data recorded in such a way that you can identify or calculate the effect size and when the studies all use the same outcome measures. This is more likely in intervention studies. Meta-analysis usually includes randomized or quasi-randomized controlled trials because these studies provide the best evidence to base decisions on. However, it should be noted that many RCTs are also at a high risk of bias. The results of the studies can then be combined statistically. You can run a meta-analysis with all studies included and then run it again without the poorer-quality studies and see what difference the omission of the studies makes.

A meta-analysis is often the end point of a systematic review and is often presented visually in a diagram referred to as a forest plot. The details of undertaking a meta-analysis need to be learnt, and an excellent source to understand this is the *Cochrane Handbook for Systematic Reviews of Interventions* (Higgins and Green 2011). This is an online handbook which is split into chapters. The book is also searchable, which makes it easier to use.

The forest plot (diagram of a meta-analysis) shown in Figure 7.1 is taken from a systematic review in which researchers reviewed studies of the mental health outcomes of people who had stopped smoking and those who continued to smoke. The aim of the study was to investigate the commonly held belief that a barrier to smoking cessation is increased stress and mental health problems. Researchers searched for studies which had examined the effect of smoking on the mental health of the participants.

A meta-analysis and forest plot were undertaken as part of the systematic review by Taylor et al. (2014), who investigated differences in the changes in mental health outcomes (for example anxiety, mixed anxiety and depression, depression, stress) in people who had stopped smoking and those who continued to smoke. They pooled the results from 26 longitudinal studies that had assessed the mental health of participants who had continued to smoke and those who had stopped smoking. They found that those who had stopped smoking had a significantly increased quality of life compared with those who continued to smoke, providing evidence that smoking cessation does not lead to additional stress, as is often claimed.

Presentation of a forest plot

If you look at the forest plot in Figure 7.2, you can see that all of the individual studies are listed on the left-hand side. The measured difference in the mean mental health score between the group who stopped smoking and the group who did not is represented by the small square in the middle of the longer line. If the data is binary, this is often presented as an odds ratio or risk ratio but in this study the data are continuous. The longer line represents the confidence intervals for the study. The confidence intervals can be taken to represent the uncertainty about the effect of stopping smoking on change in mental health. Confidence intervals are explained below.

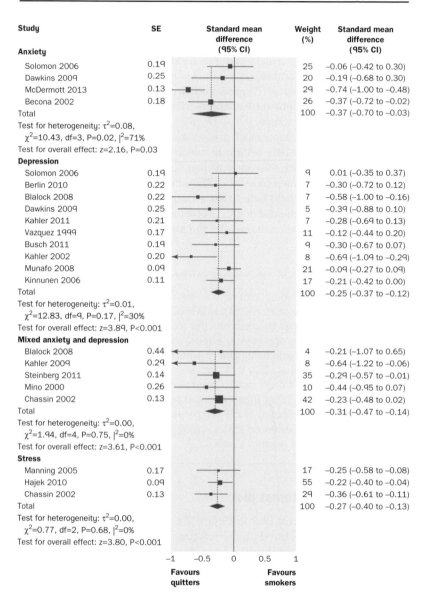

Figure 7.2 Forest plot to illustrate the changes in mental health in those who stopped smoking and those who continued to smoke, from the start of the study to follow-up (Taylor et al. 2012)

A line of 'no effect' runs down the middle of the chart. Any study where the confidence intervals cross this line indicates there is no evidence of a difference between the mental health of those who stopped smoking and those who did not so that it is a non-significant result. In this forest plot, you can see that many of the studies show benefits in the mental health of those who stopped smoking.

The weight of each study is presented as a percentage, which reflects how strongly each study contributes to the overall average effect estimate. More precise studies, those with narrower confidence intervals, contribute more weight to the overall average.

The diamond represents the average of all studies' results. The vertical points of the diamond lie on the average of all studies, and the horizontal points of the diamond represent the 95 per cent confidence interval of the average. In this study, the authors analysed each type of outcome separately (depression, anxiety and so on) and in each case the diamonds do not cross the line of no effect. Hence we can be confident that those who stopped smoking had better mental health than those who continued to smoke and that chance does not explain this. This meta-analysis shows that each individual study was generally not sufficiently precise to know this, but the average of all of them gives us much more certainty.

Confidence intervals

The confidence we can have that the sample is an accurate indication of the true population prevalence is reflected in **confidence intervals**, which give numerical limits to a 'common-sense' approach. Confidence intervals are used to estimate the confidence that the sample reflects a range within which the true score is known to lie. The smaller the interval or range, the more confident you can be that the results in the study reflect the results you would find in the larger population. Using a formula, the confidence intervals, upper and lower, are calculated. A 95 per cent confidence interval means that we can be 95 per cent sure that the true population prevalence lies between the lower and upper confidence interval. However small the confidence intervals are, if they cross the line of 'no effect' then this remains a non-significant result.

Meta-analysis training

If you are going to undertake meta-analysis then further training would be recommended. There are various courses available or it is possible to seek additional advice from a statistician or experienced reviewer. If you are going to perform a meta-analysis then consider whether it would be suitable to register your work as a Cochrane Review. Some PhD students have successfully done this but you do need to be working with a team of researchers. Initially you attempt to register your title with a specific group in Cochrane and if they want to pursue this then you get access to their editors and to their software, RevMan. RevMan is a database designed to run and report on systematic reviews. The first step is to write a protocol for the systematic review you intend to undertake, describing the methods for the main review. You would need to discuss this in detail with your supervisor.

Descriptive analysis when a meta-analysis is not possible

When you do not identify RCTs – for example, you might come across a case series with a before and after design – it is important to remember that these studies are at a higher risk of bias because they have not been designed to include blinding, randomization or other forms of comparison (although sometimes participants are compared before and after the measure). Therefore it is not possible to rule out the impact of other variables upon the outcome of the study. For example, deterioration in disease state can confound the results of before and after studies, which would be controlled for in an RCT. However, often this can be the only data available. It is still possible to use the data from the studies, but this would be described rather than used to form a summary statistic. Participant populations should be described along with whether all participants were included in the analysis. You can describe the different effect sizes, whether results were all in favour of a treatment or not and discrepancies in results. It is important to identify the limitations of the findings and the likelihood that the results will lead to the need for a definitive study in the future.

Other quantitative studies are not concerned with the measurement of an effect size, and you can also combine these using descriptive analysis. For instance, you might have findings from surveys. Once again you can describe the range of results across studies, how many responses were similar both within and across the studies. For example, some surveys may have been undertaken with all healthcare professionals whereas others may focus on just one particular group, such as nurses. You would need to decide how much this would influence the results, which may depend up the question you are asking. Indeed, you may only be interested in a small part of the survey results as they are the only part which answers your own review question. Often findings from surveys might be supported by papers which take a qualitative stance and the two can be complementary. In the next part of this chapter we will describe how to synthesize different types of data using non-statistical approaches.

Approaches to analysis and synthesis using thematic analysis

If your literature is qualitative or mixed-methods research, you are unlikely to use a statistical approach to your data analysis. A qualitative approach to data analysis will be more appropriate and there are various options you may consider. Many of these options originate from the established approaches to the analysis of qualitative data and are similar in the methods they use. We will consider a selection of these in this chapter.

Framework analysis

Framework analysis is a structured approach to data synthesis and analysis. It originated in social policy research but has been applied in a wide variety of research settings (Ritchie and Lewis 2003). The approach offers researchers the choice between a deductive approach to data analysis as described above and a more inductive approach, which we discuss later in the chapter.

In a framework approach, a set of themes are established early on in the data analysis process. These themes are usually derived from the existing literature, although they can be identified from key topics arising in the papers analysed. The defining feature of a framework analysis (Gale et al. 2013) is the creation of a matrix in which rows and columns are produced, into which the themes arising in the literature can be allocated and thereby analysed.

As with other data analysis methods which we discuss later, comparing and contrasting the results from the different research and other evidence is an essential component of this process. What distinguishes framework analysis from the inductive approaches discussed later in this chapter is the extent to which an *a priori* framework is applied to the analysis in advance. The papers in the review are then analysed against this framework. Hence this approach is largely deductive, as the themes have been identified in advance of the main analysis. However, some researchers using a framework analysis do use a more inductive approach to the development of themes and generate their themes as they arise from the papers in their review rather than, or in addition to, a pre-existing framework.

However, even when researchers follow a deductive approach, it can be advisable to consider 'open themes' in addition, to ensure that important aspects that arise in the research papers (or other evidence) are not overlooked or omitted in the pre-established themes. The *a priori* framework can be regarded as a 'draft' or provisional structure for the analysis, which can be amended as the main themes arising from the literature become apparent. Gale et al. (2013) compare the data analysis involved in framework analysis with the constant comparison approach in which constant comparisons are made across the data, which we discuss later in this chapter. Srivastava and Thomson (2009) emphasize that even when a set of *a priori* issues have been identified, it is important to maintain an open mind when identifying themes in the literature as the thematic framework is only tentative and researchers should allow the data to influence the themes and issues that arise.

For these reasons, Gale et al. (2013) emphasize that a framework approach is not aligned with an inductive or deductive approach but that this can depend on the research question and the needs of the project and the extent to which a pre-existing framework can be applied.

For a deductive approach, the themes are preselected from previous literature, but are open to refinement and amendment.

For an inductive approach, themes are generated from the data by open and unrestricted coding.

The framework analysis provides a highly structured output for summarized data and is useful when a team of researchers are working together on a project and need a consistent method of analysis. It is emphasized that the framework analysis cannot accommodate a diverse range of literature, although the approach is regarded as a flexible approach that can be adapted to many research contexts where the aim is to generate themes.

The process involved in a framework analysis is outlined by Gale et al. (2013):

- transcription
- familiarization with the data
- coding
- developing a framework
- applying a framework
- charting data into the framework
- interpreting the data

An example of a framework analysis is the review undertaken by Thorarinsdottir and Kristjansson (2014), who examined the concept of person-centred care. The reviewers searched for working definitions of how people defined person-centred care. Sixty studies were identified and from these the stages of familiarization, identifying a framework, indexing, charting and mapping the data were undertaken, followed by an interpretation. The researchers found a diversity in definitions of person-centred care that focussed on connecting, processing information and taking action.

Meta-aggregation

This is an approach to the analysis of literature which is used by those reviewing for the Joanna Briggs Institute and is based on the Cochrane approach to systematic reviews. Meta-aggregation was developed as a pragmatic strategy for analysing mainly qualitative and other data which was not appropriate for a meta-analysis. The approach is described as aggregative, or putting together, and does not explicitly encourage a re-interpretation of the literature in the review. However, the complexity of interpretative and critical understanding of the complex phenomena involved in qualitative research is acknowledged. The aim of a meta-aggregation is the product of pragmatic and generalizable statements together with recommendations for practice with an emphasis on guidance for action.

The focus of data analysis is inductive rather than the predominantly deductive approach of a framework analysis. Hannes and Lockwood (2011) identify the following process:

- The findings of studies are assembled into themes, categories and metaphors.
- Phase 1 themes are identified by the original research papers.
- Phase 2 themes are identified through further analysis.
- common themes across all papers are identified.
- Declamatory statements or line of action are identified.

Hannes and Lockwood emphasize the importance of keeping to the original data in the literature analysis and synthesis and refer to the method of constant comparison analysis as described by Lincoln and Guba (1985). Despite the reference to interpretation in a meta-aggregation,

Hannes and Lockwood (2011) emphasize that a meta-aggregation works best for the synthesis of findings where the concepts are clearly defined and well specified and where there is a clear relationship between the themes identified in the individual research paper and the final declamatory statements or lines of action. The emphasis of meta-aggregation is on the development of pragmatic lines of action which move beyond the generation of theory and can form recommendations for practice.

A meta-aggregation was undertaken by Jakimowicz et al. (2015) into patients' experience of nurse-led clinics. The researchers undertook a comprehensive search, according to pre-defined inclusion and exclusion criteria. They identified 11 papers meeting these criteria. Critical appraisal was undertaken but all of the studies were included. Significant findings were identified and aggregated into categories. Sets of statements representing the categories were produced.

Meta-ethnography

This was one of the first methods to describe the process of literature analysis and synthesis. It was described by Noblit and Hare (1988) in what has become one of the most referred-to works in the field. Although the approach was written initially for the analysis and synthesis of ethnographic studies, the authors state that it can be used with all types of qualitative research, and there are many examples of this in the literature (Campbell et al. 2011; Toye et al. 2014,). The hallmark of meta-ethnography is the focus on interpretation rather than aggregation or data summary. The approach was developed in order to avoid what the authors refer to as context stripping, incomplete and simplistic analysis and synthesis of qualitative evidence. Instead, Noblit and Hare (1988) sought an alternative approach to the analysis and synthesis of qualitative research which captured the essence and depth of the qualitative studies to be included in a review without being too 'reductionist'.

In combining the studies, the aim is to identify the relationship between the themes in all the studies, the aim of which is 'to make the obvious obvious, the obvious dubious or the hidden obvious' (Noblit and Hare 1988, p. 17).

The interpretations of literature included in a meta-ethnography are the product of the analysis and synthesis of all papers included in the review. The results of the review are interpretative and explanatory rather than 'concrete' (Noblit and Hare 1988, p. 32).

Noblit and Hare (1988) refer back to the work of Lincoln and Guba (1985), who describe the process of constant comparative analysis, a technique for the analysis of qualitative data, which is based on the work of Glaser and Strauss (1967). Noblit and Hare apply the established process of constant comparison analysis of qualitative data (raw data collected for the purposes of a qualitative research study) to the analysis and synthesis of completed qualitative research studies, so that one study can be compared against another.

This constant comparison approach is described as the basis of data analysis and synthesis in a meta-ethnography and its aim is 'a new, integrated, and more complete interpretation of findings that offers greater understanding in depth and breadth than findings from individual studies' (Bondas and Hall 2007, p. 115).

The aim of the constant comparison approach to the analysis and synthesis of qualitative research is to achieve a greater interpretative and explanatory power than a more aggregative or summative approach would allow. This process is 'one that involves opening up spaces for new insights and understandings to emerge rather than one in which totalising concepts are valued over richness and thickness of description' (Walsh and Downe 2005, p. 205).

Meta-ethnography is an example of an approach to undertaking a literature review where reviewers do not aim for a comprehensive search of the literature; a concept that we referred to in Chapter 1. Noblit and Hare (1988) argue that it may not be necessary to locate every study and that the conceptual synthesis will not be affected if five rather than ten studies are located, if they contain the same concept. The assumption here is that the ten studies will contain the same concepts as five, and that the unidentified literature will not shed new light on the literature review question. This entails a judgement which the reviewers would need to be able to defend in their written work or oral examination.

Data analysis in a meta-ethnography involves comparing the results of the different research studies included in the review. In order to do this, the results sections of the research studies are 'coded' which we describe later in this chapter so that key concepts are identified from each study and then compared to see the extent to which they can be identified in other studies. Noblit and Hare refer to this process as 'translating them into another one'. In other words, the studies are closely compared with one another. In this method, the themes identified in the results of one research paper are compared with themes that are similar in another research paper. This is referred to as reciprocal translation. Themes which illustrate opposing ideas and concepts are also compared with each other. This is referred to as refutational translation, or the analysis of deviant themes. The end result of the synthesis is the development of a line of argument, which is similar to, but less practically orientated than, the line of action developed by those undertaking a meta-aggregation.

Analysis of literature in a meta-ethnography involves:

- identifying a research question
- reading the studies
- identifying how the studies are related
- translating the studies into each other
- considering reciprocal (similar) aspects of data
- considering refutational (deviant) aspects of data
- synthesizing, or developing a line of argument

In Noblit and Hare's initial description of meta-ethnography (1988), they do not mention critical appraisal of the included studies, with the acknowledgement that all studies, irrespective of quality, will be included in the review. The argument for omitting a quality assessment is that poorer-quality studies will simply add less to the understanding of the literature as a whole rather than 'distort' the analysis. Subsequent advances in the analysis and synthesis of qualitative research have developed the role of critical appraisal, which we will discuss later in this chapter.

A meta-ethnography was the approach used by Toye et al. (2014), who investigated patients' experiences of chronic pelvic pain. In their review, the researchers did strive for a comprehensive approach to literature searching, acknowledging that this approach is not always promoted in a meta-ethnography review. They undertook a quality appraisal but did not exclude studies on the basis of quality. Key concepts were then identified and compared across the studies using a constant comparison analysis approach in order to construct a line of argument about the experience of chronic pain and the effect it had on the women's lives.

Since the publication of Noblit and Hare's (1988) seminal work, various adaptations of meta-ethnography have been developed. One of the reasons for this is undoubtedly the association of meta-ethnography with ethnographic studies. Although Noblit and Hare (1988) state that their approach can be applied to qualitative studies other than ethnography, there is an obvious assumption that, because of its name, meta-ethnography is exclusively a method for the analysis and synthesis of ethnographic studies. Consequently, many approaches to qualitative research synthesis and analysis have been developed from Noblit and Hare's original work which emphasize the analysis and synthesis of a wide range of qualitative and mixed-method approaches. These approaches are all closely based on Noblit and Hare's original work.

Thematic synthesis

Developed by Thomas and Harden (2008), this is another approach which is also closely related to the meta-ethnographic approach but which incorporates the analysis of all types of qualitative research. Thomas and Harden (2008) developed their approach from a series of studies investigating barriers and facilitators of mental health, healthy eating and physical activity in young people (Thomas et al. 2003; Harden et al. 2004) and a study to investigate pregnancy support for young people (Harden et al. 2006).

In their approach, Harden et al. (2006) refer to the 'aggregation' of studies, although in this context it is apparent that this refers to the interpretation rather than 'pooling' of qualitative studies. This illustrates that the terminology such as 'aggregation' can be used differently in different contexts and it is important to look at the meaning behind the descriptions of the methods used.

Harden et al.'s (2006) description of a thematic analysis is another example of an approach to undertaking a literature review where reviewers do not aim for a comprehensive search to the literature, but instead use a sample of relevant literature.

Thomas and Harden's (2008) approach to thematic synthesis involves the following steps:

- identifying a research question
- purposive searching, aiming for conceptual saturation rather than a comprehensive inclusion of all literature
- quality appraisal, recognizing the complexity of this
- identifying key concepts in individual studies
- developing codes and themes from the key concepts

- checking of consistency of coding/ themes between the different studies
- 'translating concepts into one another'
- generating themes; third-order interpretations

Thomas and Harden (2008) describe in detail how they coded and began to develop themes, coding each line of text according to its meaning and content (p. 3). They describe the translation of one concept into another as a key task of qualitative research synthesis, referring to the work of Britten et al. (2002) and Noblit and Hare (1988). If you compare the methods described by Noblit and Hare (1988) and Thomas and Harden (2008), it can be argued that third-order interpretations as described by Thomas and Harden (2008) are equivalent to third-order interpretations of meta-ethnography (Noblit and Hare 1988), and that the reviewers infer from the descriptive themes in order to answer the question posed by the literature review. Thus the two approaches have many similarities with some differences in the method regarding searching and critical appraisal.

For example, in the findings of their systematic review investigating the barriers and facilitators to healthy eating, Thomas and Harden (2008) found a common theme in many individual studies, that children are attracted by 'tasty' rather than 'healthy' food. In their synthesis, they were able to infer that it would be beneficial to brand fruit as 'tasty' rather than 'healthy'. They refer to this synthesis as a third-order interpretation.

A thematic synthesis was the approach used by a qualitative systematic review published by the Cochrane Collaboration, Glenton et al. (2013). In this review, researchers investigated the barriers and facilitators to the implementation of lay health workers in an attempt to improve access to maternal child health. Glenton et al. used a purposive sample of research in their review, as advocated by Thomas and Harden (2008) rather than ensuring a fully comprehensive search. A critical appraisal was undertaken and all studies were included in the review. The researchers used an *a priori* framework approach for the analysis of data, adding new themes where these were indicative from the results of the research included. The results were charted and the similarities and differences between the individual studies were summarized. The concepts were then defined and interpreted.

The researchers described the data in the studies as providing a 'thin' rather than a 'thick' description of the concepts, although their conclusions portray a comprehensive description and understanding of the role of a lay healthcare worker including the motivation for the role and how there can be tensions between those providing lay and professional care services.

Meta-synthesis

This is another approach to the analysis and synthesis of qualitative research. The term was first defined shortly before the development of meta-ethnography by Stern and Harris in 1985 and is described by Walsh and Downe (2005). Like thematic synthesis, this approach is closely related to meta-ethnography and also incorporates the principles of constant comparison analysis as described by Lincoln and Guba (1985) and Glaser and Strauss (1967). Similar to a meta-ethnography and thematic synthesis, the aims of meta-synthesis are the interpretation of qualitative research findings in order to seek new insights from a body of literature that would not be apparent from the studies viewed in isolation. Sandelowski (2004) describes the aim of meta-synthesis as providing

> *integrations that are more than the sum of the parts, in that they offer novel interpretations of findings. These interpretations will not be found in any one research report but rather are inferences derived from taking all of the reports in a sample as a whole.*
> (Sandelowski 2004, p. 1358)

The key features of a meta-analysis approach are described by Walsh and Downe (2005). Significantly, unlike meta-ethnography and thematic synthesis, Walsh and Downe (2005) recommend a comprehensive rather than a selective or purposive search strategy. As Barroso et al. (2003) recommend, 'for researchers conducting qualitative meta-synthesis projects, the ideal goal is to retrieve all of the relevant studies in a field, not just a sample of them (p. 153).

Walsh and Downe (2005) recommend that a critical appraisal of the literature is undertaken but acknowledge that this is a contested area and one that might not be easily resolved, especially with qualitative research papers, about which it can be difficult to achieve agreement as to what constitutes quality. The steps described by Walsh and Downe (2005) are:

- comprehensive search for relevant studies
- reading and re-reading of the studies
- critical appraisal of the studies
- description of how the studies are related
- analysis, in which key metaphors are compared and contrasted
- identification of themes
- organization of themes into tabulation/grid of key content
- translation of studies into each other
- identification of themes as reciprocal (similar) or refutational (contrasting)
- avoidance of 'force fitting'
- preservation of the original text to retain richness
- synthesis of translation: more refined meanings

A meta-synthesis approach was used by Noyes and Popay (2007), who synthesized research which focussed on barriers and facilitators to adherence to treatment for tuberculosis. Noyes and Popay undertook a comprehensive searching strategy, followed by a critical appraisal of the identified studies. They included all studies in their review, irrespective of their quality. On consideration, they felt that the weaker studies simply contributed less to the ongoing analysis rather than distorted the analysis. The authors describe how they brought their results together in a narrative summary and concluded that economic circumstances, material resources and individual factors affected the patient's access and compliance with treatment for tuberculosis.

Analysis and synthesis in reviews of mixed-research methods and other evidence

The seminal work of Noblit and Hare (1988) defining the process of meta-ethnography was influential in opening up debate and practice in the way in which qualitative research is brought together in a literature review. Although non-ethnographic studies were included in a meta-ethnographic study, many researchers were adamant that qualitative and quantitative research should or could not be combined in a literature review (Jensen and Allen 1996; Rogers et al. 1996). Atkins et al. (2008) also question whether different types of qualitative research can be combined in the same study, given the different philosophical positions from which they come. This approach, which might seem logical, does not take into account that many different forms of evidence might be relevant to an individual research question and that the utility of combining studies in a review might outweigh the conceptual arguments against doing so.

Further developments have seen approaches that advocate the combination of different types of research and other evidence.

Harden and Thomas (2005) argue that research questions should not be confined in their answers by the type of study but by relevance of the study to the research question and hence incorporate a range of studies in their reviews. Harden and Thomas recommend that the results of a diverse range of evidence can be analysed using a systematic approach. There are a range of methods of analysis and synthesis for literature review of mixed-method research and other evidence.

The integrative review

This is another approach that incorporates the integration of a wide range of literature in a review and has been described by Whittemore and Knafl (2005) as the

> *broadest type of research review methods, allowing for the simultaneous inclusion of experimental and non experimental research in order to more fully understand a phenomena of concern . . . Integrative reviewers may also combine data from the theoretical as well as empirical literature.*
>
> (p. 547)

The questions defined by those undertaking an integrative review can be broad, the aim of which may be to define concepts, review theories or analyse methodological issues. In an integrative review, searching is comprehensive rather than purposive, and quality appraisal is followed by data analysis. In data analysis, data are coded, ordered and categorized. Whittemore and Knafl (2005) argue that '[a] thorough and unbiased interpretation of primary sources along with an innovative synthesis of the evidence, are the goals of the data analysis stage' (p. 550).

The authors refer to the use of the constant comparison method, or other recognized qualitative approaches for data analysis. Data are compared item by item so that similar data can be compared and grouped together in order to identify themes, patterns and relationships.

Data can be displayed in a matrix or table. The method of undertaking an integrative review is described by Whittemore and Knafl as follows:

- defined question
- comprehensive (rather than purposive) search for literature
- data evaluation, quality assessment, to support the interpretation of data rather than its inclusion in the review
- data analysis: data is sorted, coded, categorized and summarized
- use of a process such as constant comparison analysis
- data displayed on a matrix, graph or chart

An example of an integrative review is that undertaken by Niela-Vilén et al. (2014), who investigated the use of Internet-based support for parents. The researchers undertook a comprehensive search and critical appraisal. No studies were omitted from the review as a result of the critical appraisal. Data analysis was undertaken following the approaches described by Whittemore and Knafl (2005). Niela-Vilén et al. (2014) concluded that Internet-based support groups provided informational support for parents which was highly accessible but which did not replace the more local support offered by other agencies.

Critical interpretative synthesis

This is a method of literature analysis and synthesis described by Dixon-Woods et al. (2006). They emphasized the need for an interpretative synthesis involving induction and interpretation and were concerned with the development of concepts and theories, rather than those already identified. For this reason, Dixon-Woods et al. (2006) suggest that an interpretative review will often avoid specifying concepts in advance of the synthesis, as discussed in Chapter 2.

Critical interpretative synthesis is based largely on Noblit and Hare's (1988) meta-ethnography, but the authors emphasize that the method can be used with a wide range of research and other evidence and hence can be more broadly applied than a meta-ethnography. Dixon-Woods et al. (2006) suggest a number of amendments to the published method of meta-ethnography. Like Noblit and Hare, they focus on the identification of a purposive sample rather than a comprehensive sample of literature. They also identified that Noblit and Hare's (1988) description of a reciprocal translational analysis tended to rely on terms already articulated in the literature and they found this to be limiting.

Dixon-Woods et al. (2006) also suggested that Noblit and Hare's (1988) description of a 'line of argument' synthesis could be better described as a 'synthesizing argument'. They acknowledge that this development is similar to Noblit and Hare's third-order constructs. Dixon-Woods et al. (2006) argue that:

> *this argument integrates evidence from across the studies in the review into a coherent theoretical framework comprising a network of constructs and relationships between them. Its function is to provide more insightful, formalized and generalizable ways of understanding phenomena.*

(p. 42)

The steps involved in a critical interpretative synthesis as outlined by Dixon-Woods et al. (2005) are:

- formulating the review question
- purposive (rather than comprehensive) searching strategy
- assessment of quality
- interpretative synthesis involving:
  - o reciprocal analysis – seeking comparisons in the literature
  - o refutational analysis – exploring differences in the literature
- producing a synthesizing argument

An example of a study using critical interpretative synthesis is that by Flemming (2010), who used this approach to interpret and develop understanding about patients' use of morphine to manage cancer pain. Flemming undertook a comprehensive search, rather than a purposive search, although she did state that if a large volume of papers had been identified, sampling would have been considered. Both qualitative and quantitative studies were identified. Critical appraisal was undertaken, although no studies were omitted from her review on the basis of this. Flemming refers to the use of a synthesis based on the work of Noblit and Hare's (1988) meta-ethnography. The results of her study included patients' concern about the use of opioids and the 'trade-offs' made by patients when they use them.

Mixed-method reviews which emphasize the role of theory

Narrative synthesis (mixed methods)

The narrative synthesis is defined by Popay et al. (2006) as a form of storytelling, relying on words and text to summarize and explain the data in a literature review. As with the meta-narrative, there is an emphasis on the role of theory within this type of review. The method was developed as a response to the need to formalize systematic review methods which were not associated with a meta-analysis. Popay et al. (2006) describe four elements to a narrative synthesis (p. 11):

- developing a theory of how the intervention works, why and for whom
- developing a preliminary synthesis of findings of included studies
- exploring relationships in the data
- assessing the robustness of the synthesis

Popay et al. (2006) define the process of a narrative synthesis as:

- identification of theory
- definition of a question
- search for literature
- appraisal of the literature
- textual description of the data
- tabulation of the data
- thematic and content analysis of the data
- reciprocal translation (similarities in the data)
- refutional translation (differences in the data)

An example of a narrative synthesis is the study by Davies et al. (2014) in which the researchers reviewed the literature on the quality of care from the perspective of the family at end of life dementia care. In their review, Davies et al. (2014) acknowledge that they did not follow all the steps of a narrative synthesis and that they did not identify a theoretical model. They undertook a comprehensive search for studies and critically appraised these although none was excluded from the study on the basis of quality. They followed Strauss and Corbin's (2008) method for analysing qualitative data in grounded theory. In their review they concluded that the perceptions of quality of care were complex and difficult to define but that quality of care was associated with the relationship with the caregivers.

Meta-narrative review

The meta-narrative review draws on the work of Kuhn (1962) and is an approach to undertaking a literature review where reviewers refer to the paradigm in which the research is located in addition to the actual research study, and incorporate both the paradigm and the study findings into the review. In order that research from different research traditions in a meta-narrative approach can be incorporated, research is compared initially from within its own paradigm so that any inconsistencies within the data can be reviewed within the paradigm in which it was described. Data analysis is undertaken following the principles of qualitative data analysis as described by Denzin and Lincoln (1994). The goal of the review is to find explanations for differences in findings and recommendations made by researchers in different traditions.

The method of undertaking a meta-narrative review is described by Greenhalgh et al. (2005) as:

- planning phase
- searching stage
- mapping stage
- appraisal stage
- synthesis stage
- recommendations stage

An example of a meta-narrative review is that undertaken by Greenhalgh et al. (2005), who investigated the diffusion, spread and sustainability of innovations in health service delivery and organization. Greenhalgh et al. undertook a comprehensive search followed by critical appraisal and analysed the research findings within the context of the paradigm within which it was set. The researchers identified 13 meta-narratives that contributed to the final report, including spreading ideas and knowledge utilization.

The realist review

The aim of a realist review is the development of theory concerning why complex interventions might work. Realist reviews often use the results and ideas generated by systematic review and continue to analyse why the interventions might work rather than just accepting the findings at face value.

Given that the aim of a realist review is the generation of theory, the search for possible theories is a central component of its initial search strategy. The evidence used in a realist review is diverse as the reviewers seek out the contextual influences, such as theories that have triggered interest in the intervention, and consider the theoretical basis as well as the empirical basis for the interventions. Despite the theory-driven context of the realist review, Greenhalgh et al. (2005) identify qualitative data synthesis as outlined by Denzin and Lincoln (1994) as the guiding concept in data analysis and synthesis.

The process involved in a realist review is identified by Pawson et al. (2005) as:

- identifying the scope of the review
- searching for theories and empirical evidence
- critical appraisal
- synthesis of findings using constant comparison analysis
- conceptual summary

A realist review was undertaken by Greenhalgh et al. (2007) following the publication of a Cochrane Collaboration systematic review which identified that school meal programmes significantly improved the growth and cognitive performance of disadvantaged children. The researchers were interested in understanding which aspects of the programme worked and for whom and in what circumstances. They analysed the studies included in the systematic review using realist methods. They constructed a matrix to analyse the data concerning the nature of the experiments and any theories or mechanisms identified by the researchers as possible explanations for the success or failure of the programmes. The researchers then searched for additional theories to explain the findings. Their analysis supported the focus of school feeding programmes on disadvantaged children but recommended that in some very malnourished children the school feeding programme could focus on providing high-energy food to compensate for food withheld at home.

Common features of qualitative and mixed-method evidence analysis and synthesis

There are many approaches to the analysis and synthesis of qualitative and mixed-method research and this book refers to only a selection of those you might come across. There are many similarities between the different methods and there can often seem to be a crossover between the different approaches. Rather confusingly, you might also find that terminology is also used interchangeably.

The approach to searching varies according to the different review methods as does the emphasis on critical appraisal. However, for the analysis and synthesis of the research and other evidence, all of the approaches refer directly back to the qualitative approaches to data analysis and the process of constant comparison analysis as outlined by Lincoln and Guba (1985), which is based on the work of Glaser and Strauss (1967), or other qualitative methodologists such as Denzin and Lincoln (1994).

It is this method of constant comparative analysis that forms the basis of most data analysis and synthesis in a literature review. As identified in the summaries of the different approaches given above, the common themes are:

- identifying themes in the data
- comparing themes across the different data
- synthesis of the themes and the development of an argument

Given the frequent reference to the method of constant comparison in the discussion of the analysis and synthesis of qualitative and mixed method in a review, we have included a detailed summary of the approach as an illustration of the way of analysing qualitative and mixed-methods research in a review.

The constant comparative analysis method

The constant comparative analysis method is widely used in the analysis of qualitative data in grounded theory but is also used in the analysis of other qualitative research projects. It is also the basis of many approaches to the analysis and synthesis of qualitative and mixed-methods literature reviews.

Given the influence of this approach on the analysis and synthesis of qualitative and mixed-method literature reviews, we will describe it in some detail here. When the constant comparative method is used to analyse literature in a review, the relevant sections of the research paper (usually the results) or other evidence are coded. Initially provisional outline codes are identified which will be developed once the data analysis is under way. Data are coded with outline codes, which are used to create broader categories. As new data are coded, these either make up a new code or fit into an existing category.

Data which have been assigned similar codes are grouped together, and these groupings form provisional categories with provisional descriptions. Lincoln and Guba (1985) describe this process as one in which researchers 'describe the category property . . . that can ultimately be used to justify the inclusion of each that remains assigned to the category as well as provide a basis for later tests of replicability and to render the category set internally consistent' (p. 347).

Subsequent coding is used to create new categories or to fit into existing categories. As each unit of analysis is coded and allocated a category, the description of the category and the content of the category are re-examined to determine the appropriate allocation of the new unit of analysis. A new or existing piece of data could be redeployed if it does not fit with the emerging category or the description of the category could be amended. As the process continues, the new additional codes may not add to the creation of new categories but refine those in existence.

Lincoln and Guba (1985) claim that 'it is this dynamic working back and forth that gives the analyst confidence that he or she is converging on some stable or meaningful data set. The test is two edged, both exposing the incident and category to searching criticism' (p. 342).

Thomas and Harden (2008) argue that using this constant comparison method, the findings are broken down and interrogated. Themes are derived via constant comparison analysis that goes back and forth until a robust set of themes emerge.

Step 1: coding your literature

The first step is to begin to code your data. This is the start of the process of identifying 'themes' from results of each study that you have. To start this process of coding, go directly to the results section of each paper and re-read this section. If your paper is discussion only, then go to the general discussion section of the paper.

If you have predominantly empirical research papers, then go through the main findings and consider how you might describe the findings the researchers present. You can use the terms used in the paper or you can paraphrase the findings in your own words. These descriptions will become the initial codes that you use to describe your data. If you have mainly discussion papers or other reports, you can allocate themes to the main discussion points.

Your codes are generated from the main findings or results of a paper; each research paper is likely to contain several codes which you can then combine with the codes from other papers. When you allocate codes to the results of the different papers, try to think of words that summarize the main point that is made in that particular section. You might choose to annotate the paper using a highlighter pen to identify the themes. Go through all your papers undertaking this method until you have assigned a code to all the appropriate results/discussion sections of the papers.

There is a variety of software that can assist you in doing this, or alternatively you can complete this analysis on hard copies of the papers. It is important to remember that computer software packages for the non-statistical analysis of literature do not do the analysis for you – they only assist you in organizing and handling the data.

Example literature review question: *What are the experiences and perceptions of the patients and nurses of the bedside handover?*

Below is an extract of the results of a study by Sand-Jecklin and Sherman (2013) in which the researchers used a mixed-method approach to investigate patients' experience and perceptions of the bedside handover, following implementation of this approach to communication about patient care. Possible initial coding is indicated in bold.

Independent T test comparisons revealed significantly higher scores (from patients) post implementation (of bedside handover) on 2 items: 'made sure I knew who my nurse was' **(introduction of nurse/patient)** and 'include in shift report' **(involvement in care)** . . . patients were invited to add narrative comments on the post implementation survey. Of the 251 comments, 102 (42%) were positive, whereas 24 (10%) indicated that nursing staff did not use bedside report, used it inconsistently or used it only to introduce the oncoming nurse . . .

Nurses were asked to respond narratively in a formative evaluation of bedside report, one month post implementation. The most frequent response to the question asking what is going well with bedside report included the following: 'checks of intravenous medication and safety,' **(assisting nursing duties)** 'introduction of oncoming staff' |**(introduction of nurse/patient)** 'assessment of patient status' **(assisting nursing duties)** and 'able to see patients earlier in the shift' **(assisting nursing duties) and (introduction of nurse/patient)** . . . . In addition, some nurses stated that bedside report 'improves accountability' and 'increases patient involvement' **(involvement in care)**.

(Sand-Jecklin and Sherman 2013, p. 190)

Below is another extract from a study by Jeffs et al. (2013), in which researchers undertook a qualitative study to explore nurses' experiences of the bedside handover. Possible initial coding is indicated in bold.

The first theme reflects how study participants described that bedside shift reporting provided an opportunity for nurses to check and clarify information **(assisting nurses duties)** relating to the status and care planning needs of patients. In some cases, by being able to check and clarify information, nurses and patients were able to identify, intercept and correct potential and actual errors in care **(assisting nursing duties)**. Several of the nurses described the value of being able to check and clarify the care plan and patient care needs with the outgoing nurse and patient. By being able to interact with them **(introduction of nurse/patient**; on further reflection code changed to **enhancing relationship between nurse and patient)** the incoming nurse was able to ask questions about missing information and determine how much the patient was being informed by other care providers about the care plan. The opportunity for patients to ask questions during the shift reporting process **(involvement in care)** was also perceived positively by many nurses.

(Jeffs et al. 2013, p. 229)

Step 2: developing themes

As you read through the results of all the papers, you will identify more codes and you will begin to see how these codes fit together into potential themes. It is useful to tabulate the emerging themes and the papers they have been identified in. You will see that some of the themes arise in all papers and that some arise in only some of the papers.

There are different ways to manage this process:

- Some people 'cut and paste' the data from their papers into themes so that they capture the entire content of the results within each theme – do keep a second copy of the paper for reference if you use this approach. This can be a good way to proceed if you like to work visually.
- Others transcribe the theme onto an electronic document so that all the extracts about each theme are grouped together electronically – if you use this approach, remember to give as much detail and avoid summarizing the data so that you retain a full description.

It is advisable to keep the original documents to hand at this point – do not put them to one side as you will need to refer back to them to check for accuracy of the themes you are developing.

Once you have allocated all the findings in the papers into themes, you need to merge all the data which have been allocated the same theme.

It is often useful to display the results of your data analysis visually on a chart such as the one presented in Table 7.1. You can then begin to see a picture emerge about the different codes and themes as they are described in your papers. Be prepared to reconsider the names of the codes and the themes and to move data around from one theme to another as your understanding of your data increases.

Step 3: naming your themes

As you continue to develop your themes, you will need to consider a provisional name for the themes as they develop. It is important to emphasize that the names of the themes are provisional at this stage. As you continue to look at the results of the papers and your understanding of the data develops, you may re-name your themes more appropriately.

Step 4: comparing the themes

The next step is to revisit each theme and check two things:

- Have you got the 'best fit' name for the theme?
- Do all the individual codes fit into the theme?

Table 7.1 Chart displaying qualitative themes

Author/date	Introduction of nurse/ patient	Assisting nursing duties	Involvement in care	Enhance relationship between nurse and patient
Sand-Jecklin and Sherman (2013)	√	√	√	
Jeffs et al. (2013)	√	√	√	√

Lincoln and Guba (1985, p. 342) describe how this 'dynamic working back and forth' gives the researcher confidence that the development of themes is robust and open to scrutiny.

It is at this point that the similarities and differences in the findings of your review will begin to emerge. Look closely at the themes you are developing and begin to consider how they are linked together. This is why it is important to keep the original documents near to hand as you may need to refer back to them to check the information or to seek further information that becomes required as your analysis progresses. If you have 'cut and pasted' the results from the original papers and grouped these together into themes you can refer back to the original sources easily. If you have compiled the themes electronically, make sure you refer back to the original sources so that you get the full meaning of the data. You will find that you have further questions that you want to ask of the papers you have and will need easy access to them.

It is frequently recommended that two or three people code each paper in order to generate maximum insight about the meaning of the paper. Unless you are working on a large funded project, this is not always possible; however, you might find it useful to discuss this process with your project supervisor or ask a friend or colleague to look over your ideas. If you do, remember to write this up in your methods section.

Step 5: consider the impact of poorer-quality studies on your themes

This is where you refer back to your critical appraisal. You will give more weight to the research that provides stronger evidence than to a weaker paper and this is why critical appraisal is important.

> **What is the impact of poorer-quality research in your literature review?**
>
> Thomas and Harden (2008) suggest that a sensitivity analysis will help you to determine the impact of weaker studies in your literature review. Just as, in a meta-analysis, researchers sometimes do the statistics with and without the weaker studies, this is also possible within a thematic analysis. If you analyse your literature including and excluding a weaker study, you can identify the impact that the weaker study has in a particular theme. Thomas and Harden argue that, often, poorer-quality studies will simply contribute less to the ongoing analysis, rather than distort it.

Step 6: consider the extent to which all your data are consistent

You might find that you have individual themes that do not support each other. The first thing to do is to consider the context of each paper from which the theme arose, together with the strengths and limitations of the research approaches undertaken. You need to return to your original critical appraisal of each paper at this point, as you need to re-assess the strength of the evidence in addressing your particular question. The rationale behind a review is that all the relevant literature is reviewed so that you can see each piece of literature in the context of the other available literature, and that differences and similarities in the results can be compared.

When you encounter literature that presents a different picture to that given by the previous literature you examined, it is important to document this carefully. Describe the differences in results and do not attempt to hide these in order to make your results appear to be more coherent. If all the data suggest different things, document this and say that you cannot reach firm conclusions from the data that you have.

You can also compare the results of research reports with non-research papers in this way, but again the contexts of both must be fully acknowledged. For example, a discussion paper by a leading expert might argue one point, but this point may not be borne out in the actual research studies that have addressed the same issues. You are likely to find research reports that contradict the opinion of an expert in the research topic area and vice versa.

Step 7: use interpretation to explain the results

Remember that this is your analysis – be creative, but do be sure that you can justify the names of the themes and the relevant inclusion of data from the original studies. At the end of this process you should have a firmed-up set of themes with names that convey the meaning of the data within them.

The importance of clarity about the method of analysis and synthesis used

In a review of methods of analysis undertaken in a literature review, Hannes and Macaitis (2012) identified a variety of approaches but also a lack of clarity about the approach that had been used. They (2012) observed that even when those undertaking a literature review had specified a named approach to analysis (for example the approach adopted by Noblitt and Hare (1988) in their meta-ethnography), a wide range of adaptations were found and many literature reviews showed no compliance with the method identified. Meta-ethnography was the most popular method of data analysis (Hannes and Macaitis 2012). Thematic analysis, as described by Thomas and Harden (2008), was also popular but sometimes lacked a definite procedure (Dixon-Woods et al. 2005, Hannes and Macaitis 2012).

The terminology used in different publications will vary. For example, Walsh and Downe (2005) and Benza and Liamputtong (2014) describe Noblit and Hare's (1988) meta-ethnography approach as a meta-synthesis.

The methods undertaken in different literature reviews will also vary. For example, not all publications which describe adherence to a method of thematic synthesis incorporate purposive sampling: for example, Satink et al. (2013) and Papadopoulou et al. (2013) both refer to a comprehensive approach to searching in their reviews.

At post-graduate level it is important to strive for a sound and rigorous methodological approach and to avoid merging approaches without a clear rationale. So we would advise you to adhere to one of the approaches we discuss in this book.

In summary

For all approaches, you will find that when you undertake a detailed systematic analysis and synthesis of the data from your literature, your findings will be displayed in a format whereby comparisons across studies can be made more easily. This can be quantitatively, such as a meta-analysis, or qualitatively, using a form of thematic analysis. Broadly speaking, there are two possible positions from which you may approach your analysis and synthesis of literature:

• meta-analysis or description of statistical data
• thematic analysis of qualitative or mixed methods

If your data is quantitative, you may consider undertaking a meta-analysis or a summary of the findings using descriptive statistics. We have referred you to further texts in order to do so. If you have qualitative data, mixed methods or a mixture of research and other evidence, you are likely to analyse and synthesize your data using one of the approaches we have discussed in this chapter. We have given the reference to the full text of the papers or books in which these approaches are fully discussed and we recommend that you access these when you have identified which approach you will be using. Whichever approach you use, it is important that you can describe and justify your rationale for adopting this approach.

Many of the qualitative and mixed-method approaches refer back to the seminal work of Glaser and Strauss (1967) and hence we have outlined a method of constant-comparison analysis to use in your review as a guide to qualitative or mixed-method analysis.

Using all of the approaches, undertaking a detailed analysis and synthesis enables you to see the strengths and weaknesses of studies and to highlight key findings. You can then start to develop arguments and generate critical understanding of the findings through a narrative report or section, which we will discuss in the next chapter.

Key points

• There is a wide variety of approaches to the analysis and synthesis of literature in your review.
• Some use a quantitative or statistical form of data analysis.
• Others use a qualitative or mixed-methods approach to data analysis.

- There are differences in the approach to searching and critical appraisal in the qualitative and mixed-method approaches.
- All of the qualitative and mixed-method approaches use a constant-comparison analysis approach.
- It is important that you identify and justify which approach is appropriate for your study.

8

How do I write up my literature review?

In this chapter we will discuss:
- *the overall presentation of your literature review*
- *how to present your review for publication*

At this stage, you will have completed a comprehensive search, data extraction, critical appraisal and analysis of the research and other evidence that constitutes your review. It is a well-established principle that research reviews are considered 'research of research' and should have the same standard of rigour as empirical research (Whittemore and Knafl 2005). Therefore, it is important that you consider that your literature review is a research study in its own right and should be presented as such. This will enable you to demonstrate that you have taken a systematic and comprehensive approach and will help you prepare your review for publication, if this is one of your aims. Given the time and effort you have invested in your literature review, we would advise that you seek to publish it.

You need to consider how you will present your review so that it is sufficiently succinct but demonstrates the detail with which you have engaged with the literature and undertaken the analysis and synthesis. Most research studies are presented in the conventional style of Introduction, Methods, Results and Discussion, which is sometimes described using the acronym IMRAD (Sollaci and Pereira 2004). If you look at the presentation of many published literature reviews, especially systematic reviews, you will see that they usually follow this structure, and adherence to this structure is generally agreed to be a feature of a good-quality literature review within health and social care (Aveyard and Sharp 2013).

The way in which you present your review will depend on the role it plays in your post-graduate project (Table 8.1). Your review will either be a standalone project, in which the results of your literature review are the main results of your project and will summarize what we know about the research question, or your review might be supportive to a larger empirical study in which case the results will demonstrate a gap in the knowledge which justifies your subsequent empirical research study. As discussed previously, however, these differences tend to be subtle and what is important is that you present your review in an appropriately structured way, with reference to the IMRAD acronym as discussed above.

If the review forms the main part of your thesis then you are likely to have a much larger word count for it than if it forms only one chapter. However, all reviews need to highlight the gaps in research evidence and the need for further research.

The structure of your literature review

In the sections below, we have discussed the individual sections of your literature review and the content you would expect to include. The information below is a guide only and you are advised to follow the specific criteria provided by your academic institution.

Table 8.1 Reflecting on the purpose of your literature review

Your literature is likely to fall into one of these categories, although sometimes the distinction might not be as clear as we have shown here.	Your literature review is a standalone study. The aim of your review is to answer (or partially answer) your literature review question.	Your literature review is supportive to a subsequent empirical study. The aim of your review is to identify gaps in knowledge that lead on to your empirical study.

Introduction and background

In your introduction, you need to explain the literature review question you are going to answer and clarify the purpose of your review and the role it plays in your project, as summarized in Table 8.1. You also need to define the key terms that you will be using. If there is a recent concept analysis of any of the key terms you use, it would be useful to draw upon this. While it is important to explain and justify your literature review question, it is important not to answer it in your introduction. Therefore it is important to avoid reference to the papers that you have identified from your search that address your literature review question. You may include a background chapter in which you set the study in context. You may draw on this again in the discussion chapter. If you are doing a systematic review as part of a PhD thesis, much of this might have been discussed in a separate section and does not need to be repeated.

Methodology and method

In your methodology, you will discuss your rationale for following the approach to the literature review you have selected. So, for example, if you have undertaken a systematic review with meta-analysis, you need to explain why this approach was appropriate. Alternatively, if you undertook a meta-ethnographic study, you need to explain the rationale for this. In the following methods section, the steps you undertook to complete your literature review including your search strategy, data extraction, critical appraisal, analysis and synthesis will be included. Your method section is likely to read like a recipe – explaining exactly what you did. This helps to make the review transparent and reassures the reader that you have been comprehensive and systematic in your method. Remember to refer directly to your literature review question. If you have more than one literature review question, you need to explain each review separately. If you have written up the methods in a separate protocol, you might consider summarizing this in your thesis but including the full protocol in an appendix.

Search strategy

Your search strategy needs to be clearly documented in your methods section so that the marker or reader of your work could replicate this if necessary. In fact, in some cases this might be a part of the assessment strategy. You need to document all the key terms and synonyms you used, how you combined these using Boolean operators, how you used truncation and controlled subject headings. The overall aim is to demonstrate to the reader that you have included all the key terms that could be reasonably expected and that you have not omitted terms which would make your review incomplete. It is useful to include a PRISMA diagram to demonstrate the process you followed, including the total number of papers identified, how decisions were made about these papers, how many duplicates there were, how many papers you read in full, as discussed in Chapter 4.

Data extraction

The way in which you undertook data extraction needs to be documented in your methods section. You should include a copy of the data extraction tool you developed and used for your review question. You should also include a completed data extraction tool in the appendix of your literature review.

Critical appraisal

Your approach to critical appraisal should be discussed in your methods section. You should also discuss the use of any critical appraisal tools used in the study and why these were chosen. If you did not use a specific tool, you can explain your rationale for this. It can be helpful to include a completed example of a critical appraisal tool in your appendix.

Analysis and synthesis

Your approach to the analysis and synthesis of literature should be described in your methods section. As we have discussed throughout this book, there is a wide variety of possible methods of data analysis and synthesis, and it is important that you can justify the approach you have taken and provide a rationale as to why it is appropriate for your study. Given the complexity of approaches and discussion of approaches, you are advised to refer directly to the original authors who developed or are developing the methods you have used for your analysis and synthesis of the literature. If you have amended the methods, then it is important to document what you have done and why.

Results

Your results need to be clearly presented, as you would expect the results of a research study to be.

It is useful to commence the presentation of your results with an overview of your papers. This can include the geographical areas they arise from, the methods they used, the dates of publication and so on.

The presentation will depend on the approach you used to analyse and synthesize your literature. Results of a meta-analysis can be clearly displayed in a forest plot. Results from a qualitative or mixed-method approach can be presented visually in a chart or matrix, but this chart also needs to be accompanied by a clear description of the data or literature from which this chart is compiled. This should be a summary rather than a list of individual papers. Hence your chart or matrix is likely to be followed by a detailed discussion of all the themes made reference to in the chart. Consider how the findings relate to each other and why different findings might have arisen. Different populations, contexts, interventions and methods of measurement might have affected the findings of the studies.

If you have found a variety of outcome measures which were difficult to make sense of, you need to explain how this has affected the results or findings of your review. It is useful to describe the way in which the interventions and outcome measures were different. For example, if an intervention was specialist care, then you can describe what this meant in each paper. This is important as it enables you to demonstrate your skills of critical appraisal – otherwise you are just reporting the results of the work of others in an uncritical way.

It is useful to compare and contrast the data which make up your themes, where the themes support each other (reciprocal themes) and where themes do not support each other (refutational themes). If word limits permit, it is also useful to give a short summary of the way in which you used the critical appraisal within your analysis. You might have analysed the literature both with and without the weaker studies in order to determine the effect of including weaker studies. You may have included only the methodologically strongest studies. It is important to discuss your reasons for the decisions you made.

Discussion

The final stage of your literature review is to bring your whole project together. This involves reflecting on your results and the way you can relate these to the literature review question and to a wider context.

This means that you have to interpret the meaning of your results and the implications they have on your project as a whole and your area of practice where appropriate. This needs to be set in the context of the limitations of what you have done. You also need to include a discussion of how your project has contributed to knowledge and theoretical understandings. Finally, you are likely to make recommendations for future research and practice. Although you are at the end of the literature review process, it is important not to rush this final section; it is your opportunity to shine and demonstrate creativity.

The following suggested structure is a guide based on the work of Doherty and Smith (1999) and Drotar (2009) regarding how to discuss the findings of a research project. It is suggested that you follow this structure when writing up your discussion and attend to each of the following points.

- statements of findings
- strength and limitations of your study
- discussion of your findings
- recommendations and implications for practice or policy or further research

The emphasis in your discussion section will depend on whether your literature review is a standalone study – in which case your discussion will seek to summarize what you have found out about your question – or whether it is a pre-requisite to a larger study – in which case you will be highlighting the gaps in knowledge and hence the need for further research (Table 8.2).

Table 8.2 Differences between the discussion section in a 'standalone' and 'main study' literature review

Your main project is an empirical study (for example PhD or master's-level project).	Your discussion will focus on the extent to which you have been able to answer your literature review question with the available literature.
Your main project is a standalone literature review (for example a master's level project).	Your discussion will focus on the next stage of your project – including how your literature review has highlighted the need for further research and a gap in the knowledge related to your research question.

Statement of findings

The findings from your literature review should be summarized, to emphasize the new knowledge your review has generated. This should be a concise summary, rather than a repetition of the details of your results section. If possible, you should attempt to summarize your findings in one or two sentences. This is only possible at the end of a study when you have done a thorough analysis and synthesis of your literature. You will not be able to 'capture' a concise and accurate summary until you have completed your analysis and synthesis.

At this point, it is appropriate to make generalizations about your findings. For example, 'most social workers were happy to undertake additional duties; however …'. You need to ensure that your generalizations convey the meaning of your findings and you need to capture the meaning of your results in a few sentences. You are likely to require several attempts at the wording of this before you communicate succinctly the meaning of your findings. Try different ways, look objectively at the meaning of what you have written and consider whether you have captured the essence of your results in these sentences. A lack of clarity about your findings often indicates a lack of clarity about your project as a whole.

You can also comment on the type of methods used in the papers, the characteristics of the groups of participants involved in the studies and what this says about the literature you included. If all the research papers you include are surveys, you might want to comment on the relevance of this to your project. Alternatively, if all the research papers are focussed on the perspective of the patient or client rather than the health or social care professional, you might want to comment on this.

Some theoretical reflections are useful too. If all of your papers refer to a particular theoretical perspective, this should be commented on. For example, you might find that all your papers refer to the attachment theory of Bowlby rather than to other theories of child development.

Strengths and limitations of your study

It is important to acknowledge the strengths and limitations of your literature review. This is because it acknowledges to the reader the drawbacks to your research and enables the results to be placed in context. In the same way as you have undertaken a critical appraisal of the information upon which your literature review is based, it is also necessary to undertake a critical appraisal of your own work.

You can emphasize what you have done to enhance the rigour of your study. Discuss the involvement of colleagues or your supervisor in the data selection, extraction, analysis and synthesis stages of your project if appropriate.

You can also emphasize what you could have done to enhance the rigour of the study. There may have been additional resources that would have enabled you to undertake a more detailed review. For example, additional finances might have enabled you to employ the assistance of other researchers who would have aided you in the search, critique and bringing together of the literature.

You can also mention what you have learnt from undertaking this research process and how you would approach a similar study in the future.

Discussion of your findings

The discussion of your findings can be one of the hardest sections to write. Until this point, you have followed a systematic and logical process that has resulted in the presentation of the results of your study. Now is the time for some creativity to enter your work and to consider what your results or findings really mean in relation to your literature review question and the purpose of your review. Discussing your findings is therefore both an art and a science.

In order to do this, you need to look at your work critically, from different perspectives and with fresh eyes. If you can take a break from your review for a few days, you might consider your findings in a different light. Talk to others about your findings and their possible implications. It might be helpful to forget the detail for a moment, and consider the most important thing that your work has demonstrated: the aspects that you would most like to share with others. This should relate to the aspects of your findings that are most important for answering your research question.

While it is important to emphasize that there is an interpretative and creative element to your literature review, it is also important to emphasize that your literature review must reflect the findings and themes you developed. Do not be tempted to exaggerate your findings so that your argument flows better. This will be identified by those who examine your work, and your findings may be discredited. If your results are inconclusive it is important to restate this rather than try to make the results appear to show something that they do not. Be honest about what you have found; remember that finding little evidence about your literature review question is a useful finding in itself.

If your literature review is a pre-requisite to an empirical study, finding minimal literature provides a justification for your further research and the development of theories.

On the other hand, you do need to provide some interpretation of your findings and make your own judgement on them. There is little point to a discussion section if you merely repeat the main findings of the study and do not exercise any judgement or interpretation of the findings (Skelton and Edwards 2000).

The main aim of your discussion of your themes is to start focussing outwards and begin to consider how the main themes you have identified relate to the wider context in which your literature review or research question is located. There are three main ways in which you can begin to compare your findings to a wider context, considering related research, policy or theory.

Integrating your results and discussion

We have suggested that, if you use the IMRAD structure for your presentation of your literature review, the results and discussion will be two separate sections. However, some researchers prefer to discuss their findings immediately after they have presented them. In this way, the theme and the discussion are read consecutively so the reader can keep the flow of the argument. If you opt to present your results and findings this way, it is important to inform the reader that this is your intention and also to ensure that your discussion does not get 'mixed up' with your results.

Relating your themes to further research

You might consider relating your themes to research in other related areas. For example, if your literature review focussed on a certain group of patients or clients, you could discuss your findings in the light of the findings of research that relate to a different group of patients or clients. If your literature review question concerned what it is like for homeless people to access medical or social care services, you might compare your findings with the experience of other 'hard to reach' groups. In order to do this, you will need to do some additional literature searches to identify papers that shed light on the topic of the literature review question when it is related to other areas. The detail in which you do this will depend on the level to which you are studying.

Relating your themes to relevant policy

You might consider relating your themes to other policy to see whether the findings of your review are in line with current policy. For example, if your literature review focussed on administration of medications and your results indicated that patients/clients prefer to administer their own medication while in hospital, you might compare how this finding fits in with policy on the self-administration of medication.

Relating your themes to relevant theories

You might consider relating your themes directly back to the theories you have identified at the start of your project or to new theories which you have come across as you have undertaken your review. For example, if your review focussed on what motivates people to lose weight, or to change any aspect of their behaviour, you can compare your findings with the current theories of behaviour change. You can also comment on the way in which your review has highlighted assumptions or problems with existing theories.

Recommendations for further research and practice

If your literature review is a standalone review, you should be able to identify some clear recommendations for practice and further research. Remember that these arise from your own original work and so you can be bold about the assertions you make. It is useful to give examples from your review to illustrate why the recommendations have been made. If your results are inconclusive, then you are likely to suggest that further research is needed. It is important to consider the way in which recommendations are made, according to your level of study. Recommendations can be listed clearly as bullet points with accompanying rationale or you may consider a more in-depth approach to the presentation and discussion of your recommendations.

Dissemination and publication

One of the obvious benefits of taking a systematic approach to your literature review is the possibility of publication of your work. Presenting your review as a study in its own right will emphasize the importance of your review and any subsequent studies that follow on. Publication of your literature review will bring credibility to your overall project and the comments from the reviewers will provide you with an additional source of feedback. The level of rigour with which you have approached your review will indicate where your review can be published. The example we provided in Chapter 5 on the management of pleural effusion (Table 5.2) was submitted for publication by the Cochrane Collaboration (Clive et al. 2013). This was because it entailed a highly rigorous method, incorporating a team of reviewers at different stages of the project. The other example in Chapter 5 on the perception of services of those experiences a life-limiting illness (Table 5.3) was submitted to a specialist palliative care journal. The rigour of this study was commented on as there was only one reviewer involved in the review process.

As a general principle, it is advisable to consult the publication guidelines for any journal to which you might submit. We advise that you do this at your earliest opportunity as you can then write with the intention of publication in this journal. Remember that different journals accept different types of literature review. The extent to which you can show rigour in the methods undertaken in your review will affect your chance of publication. Those journals with the highest impact are likely to require that you have searched on multiple databases, involved colleagues or peers in different stages of the review as discussed in Chapters 4 and 5, and presented a PRISMA checklist to demonstrate that you have followed the recognized stages of a systematic review. In addition to rigour in the methods used, you also need to demonstrate the impact and usefulness of the review, so the discussion section is vital.

Above all, you need to be concise in your presentation. Journal papers are often limited to 3000–5000 words. Many are not able to print multiple tables but this might be possible in online editions. You may have to edit and summarize the main findings of your review but you can refer the reader to the full version of your project or thesis for further information.

Practical ways to enhance the presentation of your literature review

There are some straightforward practical ways that you can enhance the presentation of your work. This might sound obvious, but clearly presented work will make it easier for your examiner to award you marks. The following are some tips to help you with your presentation:

- Ask a friend or colleague to proofread your work.
- Concentrate on checking for typos.

- Return to your work after a break and read it again with fresh eyes.
- Make good use of headings and tables.
- Make sure all your references are completed.

In summary

The important point to remember is that a literature review is a study in its own right and you should usually present it as such, according to the standard scientific structure of IMRAD. Presenting your review according to this structure will also enable you to prepare your work for publication as most journals will require this structure. When you write up your methods, you need to write succinctly while not losing the detail and complexity with which you undertook your review. Your results section should be presented as a meta-analysis or a theme-based approach, with a justification for the approach you took. Your discussion needs to relate your main findings to relevant research, theories or policies. Finally, remember to summarize the extent to which your review has answered your research question or paved the way for your subsequent larger empirical study.

Key points

- Your literature review should normally be written up using the standard scientific structure, IMRAD.
- You need to give clear and succinct details about the method you undertook in your literature review, including how you searched, extracted data, and appraised and analysed your literature.
- Ensure your discussion is an accurate reflection of the results.
- Summarize your main findings in the discussion section, but briefly!
- Acknowledge the strengths and limitations of your review.
- Discuss your findings in relation to relevant research, policies or theories.
- Discuss any unanswered questions and recommendations for future research.

References

Akoberg AK (2005) Understanding randomised controlled trials. *Archives of Diseases in Childhood* 90: 840–4

Arksey H and O'Malley L (2005) Scoping studies: Towards a methodological framework. *International Journal of Social Research Methodology* 8(1): 19–32

Atkins S, Lewin S, Smith H, Engel M, Fretheim A and Volmink J (2008) Conducting a meta-ethnography of qualitative literature: Lessons learnt. *BMC Medical Research Methodology* 16(8): 21

Aveyard H and Neale J (2009) Critical incident technique, in Neale J (ed.) *Research Methods for Health and Social Care*. London. Palgrave Macmillan

Aveyard H and Sharp P (2013) *A Beginner's Guide to Evidence Based Practice*. Maidenhead. Open University Press

Balfour DJ and Fagerstrom KO (1996) Pharmacology of nicotine and its therapeutic use in smoking cessation and neurodegenerative disorders. *Pharmacology Therapy* 72(1): 51–81

Barroso J, Gollop CJ, Sandelowski M, Meynell J, Pearce P and Collins LJ (2003) The challenge of searching for and retrieving qualitative studies. *Western Journal of Nursing Research* 25(2): 153–78

Bates MJ (1989) The design of browsing and berry picking techniques for the online search interface. *Online Review* 13: 407–23

Beck CT (2009) Critiquing qualitative research. *AORN Journal* 90(4): 543–4

Benza S and Liamputtong P (2014) Pregnancy, childbirth and motherhood: A meta-synthesis of the lived experience of immigrant women. *Midwifery* 30: 575–84

Betrán AP, Say L, Gülmezoglu AM, Allen T and Hampson L (2005) Effectiveness of different databases in identifying studies for systematic reviews: Experience from the WHO systematic review of maternal morbidity and mortality. *BMC Medical Research Methodology* 5(1): 6

Bettany-Saltikov J (2012) *How to Do a Systematic Literature Review in Nursing*. Maidenhead. Open University Press

Bondas T and Hall EOC (2007) Challenges in approaching metasynthesis research. *Qualitative Health Research* 17: 113

Booth A (2008) Using evidence in practice. *Health Information and Libraries Journal* 25: 313–17

Booth A (2010) How much searching is enough? Comprehensive versus optimal retrieval for technology assessments. *International Journal of Technology Assessments in Health Care* 26: 431–5

Borgerson K (2009) Valuing evidence: Bias and the evidence hierarchy of evidence-based medicine. *Perspectives in Biology and Medicine* 52(2): 218–33

Bradshaw A (2015) Shaping the future of nursing: Developing an appraisal framework for public engagement with nursing policy reports. *Nursing Inquiry* 22(1): 74–83

Britten N, Campbell R, Pope C, Donovan J, Morgan M and Pill R (2002) Using meta-ethnography to synthesise qualitative research: A worked example. *Journal of Health Services Research and Policy* October 7(4): 209–15

Burls A (2009) What is critical appraisal? *What is...? series.* Newmarket. Haywood Medical Communications

Campbell R, Pound P, Morgan M, Daker-White G, Britten N, Pill R, Yardley L, Pope C and Donovan J. (2011) Evaluating meta-ethnography: Systematic analysis and synthesis of qualitative research. *Health Technology Assessment* 15(43): 1–164

Candy B, France R, Low J and Sampson L (2015) Does involving volunteers in the provision of palliative care make a difference to patient and family wellbeing? A systematic review of quantitative and qualitative evidence. *International Journal of Nursing Studies* 52: 756–68

Caraceni A, Hanks G, Kaasa S, Bennett MI, Bruneli C, Cherny N, Dale O, De Conno F, Fallon M, Hanna M, Haugen DF, Juhl G, King S, Klepstad P, Laugsand EA, Maltoni M, Mercandante S, Nabal M, Pigni A, Radbruch L, Reid C, Sjogren P, Stone PC, Tassinari D and Zeppetella G (2012) Use of opioid analgesics in the treatment of cancer pain: Evidence-based recommendations from the EAPC. *Lancet Oncology* 13(2): e58–e68.

Centre for Reviews and Dissemination (2008) *Systematic Reviews: CRD's Guidance for Undertaking Reviews in Health Care.* York. University of York

Chandler J and Hopewell S (2013) Cochrane methods: Twenty years experience in developing systematic review methods. *Systematic Reviews* 2(76). Cochrane Methodology Anniversary Series. Available at www.systematicreviewsjournal.com/content/2/1/76 (accessed 23 September 2015)

Chapman AL, Morgan LC and Gartlehner G (2009) Semi-automating the manual literature search for systematic reviews increases efficiency. *Health Information and Libraries Journal* 27: 22–7

Citrome L, Moss SV and Graf C (2009) How to search and harvest the medical literature: Let the citations come to you, and how to proceed when they do. *International Journal of Clinical Practice* 63(11): 1565–70

Citrome L, Moss SV and Graf C (2011) How to search and harvest the medical literature: Let the literature come to you and how to proceed when they do. *International Journal of Clinical Practice* 26(1): 26–31

Clark AM, King-Shier KM, Spaling MA, Duncan AS, Stone JA, Jaglal SB, Thompson DR and Angus JE (2013) Factors influencing participation in cardiac rehabilitation programmes after referral and initial attendance: Qualitative systematic review and meta-synthesis. *Clinical Rehabilitation* 27(10): 948–59

Cleary M, Horsfall J and Hayter M (2014) Data collection and sampling in qualitative research: Does size matter? *Journal of Advanced Nursing* 70: 473–5

Clive A, Bhatnagar R, Preston NJ, Jones HE and Maskell N (2013) Interventions for the management of pleural effusions. *Cochrane Collaboration Protocol*

Cochrane AL (1972) *Effectiveness and Efficiency: Random Reflections on Health Services.* London. Nuffield Provincial Hospitals Trust

Cochrane AL (1979) 1931–1971: Critical review, with particular reference to the medical profession, in *Medicines for the Year* 2000. London. Office of Health Economics

Cooke A, Smith D and Booth A (2012) Beyond PICO: The SPIDER tool for qualitative evidence synthesis. *Qualitative Health Research* 22(10):1435–43

Cottrell S (2011) *Critical Thinking Skills.* London. Palgrave Macmillan

Coughlan M, Cronin P and Ryan F (2007) Step by step guide to critiquing research. Part 1: quantitative research. *British Journal of Nursing* 16(11): 658–63

Davies N, Maio L, Rait G and Iliffe S (2014) Quality end-of-life care for dementia: What have family carers told us so far? A narrative synthesis. *Palliative Medicine* 28(7): 919–30

Denzin NK (2009) The elephant in the living room: Or extending the conversation about the politics of evidence. *Qualitative Research* 9(2): 139–60

Denzin NK and Lincoln P (1994) *Handbook of Qualitative Research.* London. SAGE Publications

Dewey J (1938) *Logic: The Theory of Enquiry.* New York. Longman Green.

Dixon-Woods M, Agarwal S, Jones D, Young B and Sutton A (2005) Synthesising qualitative and quantitative evidence: A review of possible methods. *Journal of Health Services Research and Policy* 10: 45–53

Dixon-Woods M, Cavers D, Agarwal S, Annandale E, Arthur E, Harvey J, Hsu R, Katbamna S, Olsen R, Smith L, Riley R and Suootn A (2006) Conducting a critical interpretive synthesis of the literature on access to health care of vulnerable groups. *BMC Research Methodology* 6(35)

Dixon-Woods M, Sutton A, Shaw R, Miller T, Smith J, Young B, Bonas S, Booth A and Jones D (2007) Appraising qualitative research for inclusion in systematic reviews: A quantitative and qualitative comparison of three methods. *Journal of Health Service Research Policy* 12(1): 42–7

Doherty M and Smith R (1999) The case for structuring the discussion of scientific papers. *British Medical Journal* 318: 1224–5

Drotar D (2009) Editorial: How to write an effective results and discussion for *Journal of Paediatric Psychology. Journal of Paediatric Psychology* 34(4): 330–43

Emerson JD, Burdick E, Hoaglin DC, Mosteller F and Chalmers TC (1990) An empirical study of the possible relation of treatment differences to quality scores in controlled randomized clinical trials. *Controlled Clinical Trials* 11: 339–52

Estabrooks CA, Field PA and Morse JM (1994) Aggregating qualitative findings: An approach to theory development. *Qualitative Health Research* 4: 503–11

Fawcett J (2005) Criteria for the evaluation of theory. *Nursing Science Quarterly* 18(2): 131–5

Fielding N (2010) Elephants, gold standards and applied qualitative research. *Qualitative Research* 10(1): 123–7

Fineout-Overholt E and Johnston L (2005) Teaching EBP: Asking searchable, answerable clinical questions. *World Views on Evidence-Based Nursing* 2(3): 157–60

Finfgeld D (1999) Courage as a process of pushing beyond the struggle. *Qualitative Health Research* 9(6): 803–14

Finfgeld-Connett D (2014) Intimate partner abuse among older women: Qualitative systematic review. *Clinical Nursing Research* 23(6): 664–83

Finfgeld-Connett D and Johnson ED (2013) Literature search strategies for conducting knowledge-building and theory-generating qualitative systematic reviews. *Journal of Advanced Nursing* 69(1): 194–204

Finlayson KW and Dixon A (2008) Qualitative meta-synthesis: A guide for the novice. *Nurse Researcher* 15(2): 59–71

Flemming K (2010) Synthesis of quantitative and qualitative research: An example using Critical Interpretive Synthesis. *Journal of Advanced Nursing* 66(1): 201–17

Flemming K, Graham H, Heirs M, Fox D and Sowden A (2013) Smoking in pregnancy: A systematic review of qualitative research of women who commence pregnancy as smokers. *Journal of Advanced Nursing* 69(5): 1023–36

Ford N and Maher D (2013) Making sure that clinical trial results make a difference: Operational research and the hierarchy of evidence. *Tropical Medicine* 18(4): 504–5

Freshwater D, Cahill J, Walsh E and Muncey T (2010) Qualitative research as evidence: Criteria for rigour and relevance. *Journal of Research in Nursing* 15(6): 497–508

Gale NK, Heath G, Cameron E, Rashid S and Redwood S (2013) Using the framework method for the analysis of qualitative data in multidisciplinary health research. *BMC Medical Research Methodology* 13(117)

Gilbert R, Salanti G, Harden M and See S (2005) Infant sleeping position and the sudden infant death syndrome: Systematic review of observational studies and historical review of recommendations 1940–2002. *International Journal of Epidemiology* 34(4): 874–87

Gilbert E, Ussher J and Hawkins Y (2009) Accounts of disruptions to sexuality following cancer: The perspective of informal carers who are partners of a person with cancer. *Health* 13(5): 523–41

Giles TM and Hall KL (2014) Qualitative systematic review: The unique experiences of the nurse-family member when a loved one is admitted with a critical illness. *Journal of Advanced Nursing* 70(7): 1451–64

Glaser BG and Strauss A (1967) The constant comparative method of qualitative analysis, in *The Discovery of Grounded Theory*. Chicago. Aldine

Glenton C, Colvin CJ, Carlsen B, Swartz A, Lewin S, Noyes J and Rashidian A (2013) Barriers and facilitators to the implementation of lay health worker programmes to improve access to maternal and child health: Qualitative evidence synthesis. *Cochrane Database of Systematic Reviews* 10: CD010414

Gøtzsche PC and Nielsen M (2011) Screening for breast cancer with mammography. *The Cochrane Database of Systematic Reviews* 19(1).

Grant MJ and Booth A (2009) A typology of reviews: An analysis of 14 review types and associated methodologies. *Health Information and Libraries Journal* 26(2): 91–108

Greaves CJ, Sheppard KE, Abraham C, Hardeman W, Roden M, Evans PH, Schwarz P and the Image Study Group (2011) Systematic review of reviews of intervention components associated with increased effectiveness in dietary and physical activity interventions *BMC Public Health* 11(18): 119

Greenhalgh T (2014), @trishgreenhalgh, on Twitter 3–5 May 2014

Greenhalgh T and Peacock R (2005) Effectiveness and efficiency of search methods in systematic reviews of complex evidence: Audit of primary sources. *British Medical Journal* 331: 1064–5

Greenhalgh T, Robert G, Macfarlane F, Bate P, Kyriakidou O and Peacock R (2005) Storylines of research in diffusion of innovation: A metanarrative approach to systematic review. *Social Science Medicine* 61: 417–30

Greenhalgh T, Kristjansson E and Robinson V (2007) Realist review to understand the efficacy of school feeding programmes. *British Medical Journal* 335: 858–62

Hannes K and Lockwood C (2011) Pragmatism as the philosophical foundation for the Joanna Briggs meta-aggregative approach to qualitative evidence synthesis. *Journal of Advanced Nursing* 67(7): 1632–42

Hannes K and Macaitis K (2012) A move to more systematic and transparent approaches in qualitative evidence synthesis: Update on a review of published papers. *Qualitative Research* 12(4): 402–42

Harden A (2007) Does study quality matter in systematic reviews which include qualitative research? Paper presented at XV Cochrane Collaboration colloquium, São Paulo Brazil, 23–27 October

Harden A and Thomas J (2005) Methodological issues in combining diverse study types in systematic reviews. *International Journal of Social Research Methodology* 8(3): 257–71

Harden A, Garcia J, Oliver S, Rees R, Shepherd J, Brunton G and Oakley A (2004) Applying systematic review methods to studies of people's views: An example from public health. *Journal of Epidemiology and Community Health* 58: 794–800

Harden A, Brunton G, Fletcher A and Oakley A (2006) *Young People, Pregnancy and Social Exclusion: A Systematic Synthesis of Research Evidence to Identify Effective, Appropriate and Promising Approaches for Prevention and Support.* London EPPI-centre, Social Science Research Unit, Institute of Education, University of London

Hawker S, Payne S, Kerr C, Hardey M and Powell J (2002). Appraising the evidence: Reviewing disparate data systematically. *Qualitative Health Research* 12(9): 1284–99

Hawkins Y, Ussher J, Gilbert E, Perz J, Sandoval M and Sundquist K (2009) Changes in sexuality and intimacy after the diagnosis and treatment of cancer. *Cancer Nursing* 32(4): 271–80

Heidegger M (1962) *Being and Time*, translated by J Macquarrie and E Robinson. Oxford: Blackwell Publishing

Higgins JPT and Green S (2011) *Cochrane Handbook for Systematic Reviews of Interventions*, version 5.1.0. The Cochrane Collaboration. www.cochrane-handbook.org

Hoppe DJ, Schemitsch EH, Morshed S, Tornetta P and Bhandari, M (2009) Hierarchy of evidence: Where observational studies fit in and why we need them. *The Journal of Bone and Joint Surgery: American volume* 91 (Supplement 3): 2–9

Jakimowicz S, Stirling C and Duddle M (2015) An investigation into factors that impact patients' subjective experience of nurse led clinics: A qualitative systematic review. *Journal of Clinical Nursing* 24(1–2): 19–33

Jeffs L, Acott A, Simpson E, Campbell H, Irwin T, Lo J, Beswick S and Cardoso R (2013) The value of bedside shift reporting. *Journal of Nursing Care Quality* 28(3): 226–32

Jensen LA and Allen MN (1996) Meta-synthesis of qualitative findings. *Qualitative Health Research* 6(4): 553–60

Joanna Briggs Institute (2014) *Reviewers' Manual.* Australia

Just ML (2012) Is literature search training for medical students and residents effective? A literature review. *Journal of Medical Library Association.* 100(4): 270–6

Katrak P, Bialocerkowski AE, Massy-Westrop N, Kumar VSS and Grimmer KA (2004) A systematic review of the content of critical appraisal tools. *BMC Medical Research Methodology* 4:22

Kuhn TS (1962) *The Structure of Scientific Revolution.* Chicago. University of Chicago Press

Langenhoff JM and Schoones JW (2011) Letter to the editor in response to 'Risk factors for bladder cancer: Challenges for conducting a literature search using PubMed', *Perspectives in Health Information Management* 8(4): 1

Law M, Stewart D, Pollock N, Letts L, Bosch J and Westmorland M (1998) *Guidelines for Critical Review Form: Quantitative Studies*. Ontario. McMaster University. Available at: http://srs-mcmaster.ca/wp-content/uploads/2015/05/Guidelines-for-Critical-Review-Form-Quantitative-Studies.pdf

Leung W (2001) How to design a questionnaire. *Student BMJ* 9: 188–9

Lincoln YS and Guba EG (1985) *Naturalistic Inquiry*. Beverly Hills. SAGE Publications

Lindberg C, Fagerstrom, Sivberg B and Willman A (2014) Concept analysis: Patient autonomy in a caring context. *Journal of Advanced Nursing* 70(10): 2208–21

Lindson N (2012) Smoking reduction and nicotine preloading: New approaches to cessation. PhD thesis, University of Birmingham

Marmot MG, Altman DG, Cameron DA, Dewar JA, Thompson SG and Wilcox M (2012) The benefits and harms of breast cancer screening: An independent review. *The Lancet* 380(9855): 1778–86

Mason M (2014) The illegal drug use behaviour and social circumstances of older adult class A drug users in England. PhD thesis, Oxford Brookes University

Mattioli S, Farioli A, Cooke RM, Baldasseroni A, Ruotsalainen J, Placidi D, Curti S, Mancini G, Fierro M, Campo G, Zanardi F and Violante FS (2012) Hidden effectiveness? Results of hand-searching Italian language journals for occupational health interventions. *Occupational and Environmental Medicine* 69(7): 522–4.

Mays N, Pope C and Popay J (2005) Details of approaches to synthesis. A methodological appendix to the paper: Systematically reviewing qualitative and quantitative evidence to inform management and policy making in the health field. Ottawa and London. Canadian Health Services Research Foundation NHS Service Delivery and Organisation R&D Programme

McCormack B, Rycroft-Malone J, Decorby K, Hutchinson AM, Bucknall T, Kent B, Schultz A, Snelgrove-Clarke E, Stetler C, Titler M, Wallin L and Wilson V (2013) A realist review of interventions and strategies to promote evidence-informed healthcare: A focus on change agency. *Implementation Science* 8(107)

McKibbon KA, Wilczynski NL and Haynes RB (2006) Developing optimal search strategies for retrieving qualitative studies in PsycINFO. *Evaluations and the Health Professions* 29(4): 440–54

Merlin T, Weston A and Tooher R (2009) Extending an evidence hierarchy to include topics other than treatment: Revising the Australian 'levels of evidence'. *BMC Medical Research Methodology* 11(9): 34

Methley AM, Campbell S, Chew-Graham C, McNally R, Cheraghi-Sohi S (2014) PICO, PICOS and SPIDER: A comparison study of specificity and sensitivity in three search tools for qualitative systematic reviews. *MNC Health Services Research* 14: 579

Mulrow CD (1994) Systemic reviews: Rationale for systematic reviews. *British Medical Journal* 309: 597–9

Niela-Vilén H, Axelin A, Salantera S and Melender (2014) Internet-based peer support for parents: A systematic integrative review. *International Journal of Nursing Studies* 51(11): 1524–37

Noblit GW and Hare RD (1988) Meta-ethnography, synthesising qualitative studies, in *Qualitative Research Methods*, Volume 11. London. SAGE Publications

Noyes J (2010) Never mind the quality, feel the depth! The evolving role of qualitative research in Cochrane intervention reviews. *Journal of Research in Nursing* 15(6): 525–34

Noyes J and Popay J (2007) Directly observed therapy and tuberculosis: How can a systematic review of qualitative research contribute to improving services? A qualitative meta-synthesis. *Journal of Advanced Nursing* 57(3): 227–43

O'Mathuna DP (2010) Critical appraisal of systematic reviews. *International Journal of Nursing Practice* 16(4): 414–18

Papadopoulou C, Johnston B and Themessi-Huber M (2013) The experience of acute leukaemia in adult patients: A qualitative thematic synthesis. *European Journal of Oncology Nursing* 17: 640–8

Papaioannou D, Sutton A, Carroll C, Wong R and Booth A (2010) Literature searching for social science systematic reviews: Consideration of a range of search techniques. *Health Information and Libraries Journal* 27(2): 114–22

Papavasiliou E, Payne S, Brearley S, Brown J and Seymour J (2013) Continuous sedation (CS) until death: Mapping the literature by bibliometric analysis. *Journal of Pain and Symptom Management* 45(6): 1073–82

Pawson R, Greenhalgh T, Harvey G and Walshe K (2005) Realist review: A new method of systematic review designed for complex policy interventions. *Journal of Health Services Research and Policy* 10 (Supplement 1): 21–34

Payne SA and Turner JM (2008) Research methodologies in palliative care: A bibliometric analysis. *Palliative Medicine* 22: 336–42

Pearson A (2010) Evidence-based health care and qualitative research. *Journal of Research in Nursing* 15(6): 489–93

Peoples H, Satink T and Steultjens E (2011) Stroke survivors' experiences of rehabilitation: A systematic review of qualitative studies. *Scandinavian Journal of Occupational Therapy* 18: 163–71

Petticrew M and Roberts H (2005) *Systematic Reviews in the Social Sciences: A Practical Guide*. Oxford. Blackwell Publishing

Popay J, Roberts H, Sowden A, Petticrew M, Arai L, Rodgers M and Britten N (2006) *Guidance on the Conduct of Narrative Synthesis in Systematic Reviews*. ESRC Methods Programme. Swindon. ESRC

Pope C and Mays N (2006) Synthesising qualitative data, in *Qualitative Research in Health Care*. Oxford. Blackwell Publishing

Pope C, Mays N and Popay J (2007) *Synthesising Qualitative and Quantitative Health Evidence: A Guide to Methods*. Maidenhead. Open University Press

Preston NJ (2004) The development of a nursing intervention for the management of malignant ascites. PhD dissertation, Institute of Cancer Research, London

Prochaska JO, Norcross JC, DiClemente, CC (1994) *Changing for Good*. New York. William Morrow

Richardson WS (1998) Ask, and ye shall retrieve [EBM note]. *Evidence-Based Medicine* 3(4): 100–1

Ritchie J and Lewis J (2003) *Qualitative Research Practice: A Guide for Social Science Students and Researchers*. London. SAGE Publications

Rock S, Michelson D, Thomson S and Day C (2015) Understanding foster placement instability for looked after children: A systematic review and narrative synthesis of quantitative and qualitative evidence. *British Journal of Social Work* 45: 177–203

Rogers A, Popay J and Williams G (1996) Rationale and standards for the systematic review of qualitative literature in health services research. Paper presented at the third international interdisciplinary qualitative health research conference, Bournemouth, England

Ryan F, Coughlan M and Cronin P (2007) Step-by-step guide to critiquing research. Part 2: qualitative research. *British Journal of Nursing* 16(12): 738–44

Saba M, Diep J, Saini B and Dhippayom T (2014) Meta-analysis of the effectiveness of smoking cessation interventions in community pharmacy. *Journal of Clinical Pharmacy & Therapeutics* 39(3): 240–7

Sackett DL, Rosenberg WMC, Muir Gray JA, Haynes RB and Richardson WS (1996) Evidence based medicine: What it is and what it isn't. *British Medical Journal* 312: 71–2

Sampson FC, Goodacre SW and O'Cathain H (2014) Interventions to improve the management of pain in the emergency department: Systematic review and narrative synthesis. *Emergency Medicine Journal* e9–e18

Sand-Jecklin K and Sherman J (2013) Incorporating bedside report into nursing handoff. *Journal of Nursing Care Quality* 28(2): 186–94

Sandelowski M (2004) in Thorne S, Jensen L, Kearney MII, Noblit G and Sandelowski M, Qualitative meta-synthesis: Reflections on methodological orientation and ideological agenda. *Qualitative Health Research* 14: 1342–65

Sandelowski M, Docherty S and Emden C (1997) Qualitative metasynthesis: Issues and techniques. *Research in Nursing and Health* 20: 365–71

Satink T, Cup E, Ilott I, Prins J, Swart BJ and Nihuis-van der Sanden (2013) Patients' views on the impact of stroke on their roles and self: A thematic synthesis of qualitative studies. *Archives of Physical Medicine and Rehabilitation.* 93: 1171–83

Sayer A (2000) *Realism and Social Science.* London. SAGE Publications

Schulz KF and Grimes DA (2002) Allocation concealment in randomised trials: Defending against deciphering. *The Lancet* 359(9306): 614–18

Schulz KF, Chalmers I, Hayes RJ and Altman DG (1995) Empirical evidence of bias: Dimensions of methodological quality associated with estimates of treatment effects in controlled trials. *Journal of the American Medical Association* 273: 408–12

Seers K (2007) Evaluating complex interventions. *Worldviews on Evidence-Based Nursing* 4(2): 67–8

Shin KR, Kim MY and Chung SE (2009) Methods and strategies utilized in published qualitative research. *Qualitative Health Research* 19(6): 850–8

Sibbald B and Roland M (1998) Understanding controlled trials: Why are randomised controlled trials important? *British Medical Journal* 316(7126): 201

Skelton J and Edwards SLJ (2000) The function of the discussion section in academic medical writing. *British Medical Journal* 320(7244): 1269–70

Smiddy MP, O'Connell R and Creedon SA (2015) Systematic qualitative literature review of health care workers' compliance with hand hygiene guidelines. *American Journal of Infection Control* 43(3): 269–74

Smith ML and Shurtz S (2012) Search and ye shall find: Practical literature review techniques for health educators. *Health Promotion Practice* 13(5): 666–9

Sollaci LB and Pereira MG (2004) The introduction, method, results and discussion (IMRAD) structure: A fifty-year survey. *Journal of Medical Libraries Association* 92(3): 364–7

Spencer L, Ritchie J, Lewis J and Dillon L (2003) Quality in qualitative evaluation: A framework for assessing research evidence. *National Centre for Social Research.* Occasional papers series 2. London. Government Chief Social Researcher's Office, Cabinet Office

Srivastava A and Thomson SB (2009) Framework analysis: A qualitative methodology for applied policy research. *Journal of Administration and Governance* 4(2): 72–9

Stern P and Harrris C (1985) Women's health and the self-care paradox: A model to guide self-care readiness – clash between the client and nurse. *Health Care for Women International* (61–3): 151–63

Strauss A and Corbin J (2008) *Basics of Qualitative Research, Techniques and Procedures for Developing Grounded Theory.* Newbury Park, CA. SAGE Publications

Taylor B (2012) Couples living in twilight: A Heideggerian hermeneutic study of sexuality and intimacy in life-limiting illness. PhD thesis, Oxford Brookes University

Taylor B (2015) Does the caring role preclude sexuality and intimacy in coupled relationships? *Sexuality and Disability* 3: 365–74

Taylor B and de Vocht H (2011) Interviewing separately or as couples? Considerations of authenticity of method. *Qualitative Health Research* 21(11): 1576–87

Taylor G, McNeill A, Girling A, Farley A, Lindson Hawley N and Aveyard P (2014) Changes in mental health after smoking cessation: Systematic review and meta-analysis. *British Medical Journal* 348: g1151

Thiselton AC (2012) Reception theory, HR Jauss and the formative power of scripture. *Scottish Journal of Theology* 65: 289–308

Thomas J and Harden A (2008) Methods for the thematic synthesis of qualitative research in systematic reviews. *BMC Medical Research Methodology* 8: 45

Thomas J, Sutcliffe K, Harden A, Oakley A, Oliver S, Rees R, Brunton G and Kaanagh J (2003) *Children and Unhealthy Eating: A Systematic Review of the Barriers and Facilitators*. London. EPPI-Centre, Social Science Research Unit, Institute of Education

Thorarinsdottir K and Kristjansson K (2014) Patients' perception of person-centred participation in healthcare: A framework analysis. *Nursing Ethics* 21(2): 129–47

Thorne S, Jensen L, Kearney MH, Noblit G and Sandelowski M (2004) Qualitative meta-synthesis: Reflections on methodological orientation and ideological agenda. *Qualitative Health Research* 14: 1342–65

Thouless RH and Thouless CR (1953) *Straight and Crooked Thinking*. Sevenoaks. Hodder & Stoughton

Tong A, Sainsbury P and Craig J (2007) Consolidated criteria for reporting qualitative research (COREQ): A 32-item checklist for interviews and focus groups. *International Journal for Quality in Health Care* 19(6): 349–57

Toye F, Seers K and Barker K (2014) A meta-ethnography of patients' experience of chronic pelvic pain: Struggling to construct pelvis pain as 'real'. *Journal of Advanced Nursing* 70(12): 2713–27

Treweek S, Lockhart P, Pitkethly M, et al. (2013) Methods to improve recruitment to randomised controlled trials: Cochrane systematic review and meta-analysis. *BMJ Open* 3: e002360

Tucker JA and Roth DL (2005) Extending the evidence hierarchy to enhance evidence-based practice for substance use disorders. *Addiction* 101(7): 918–32

Wall S (2008) A critique of evidence-based practice in nursing: Challenging the assumptions. *Social Theory and Health* 6: 37–53

Wallace M and Wray A (2011) *Critical Reading and Writing for Postgraduates*. London. SAGE Publications

Walsh D and Downe S (2005) Meta-synthesis method for qualitative research: A literature review. *Journal of Advanced Nursing* 50(2): 204–11

Walsh D and Downe S (2006) Appraising the quality of qualitative research. *Midwifery* 22: 108–19

West R (2006) *Theory of Addiction.* Oxford. Addiction Press/Blackwell Publishing

Whittemore R and Knafl K (2005) The integrative review: Updated methodology. *Journal of Advanced Nursing* 52: 546–53

Whittemore R, Chase S and Mandle C (2001) Validity in qualitative research. *Qualitative Health Research* 11(4): 522–37

Wilczynski NL, Marks S and Haynes RB (2007) Search strategies for identifying qualitative studies in CINAHL. *Qualitative Health Research* 17(5): 705–10

Wiles R, Crow G and Pain H (2011) Innovation in qualitative research methods: A narrative review. *Qualitative Research* 11(5): 587–604

Wong G, Greenhalgh T, Westhorp G, Buckingham J and Pawson R (2013a) RAMESES publication standards: Realist syntheses. *BMC Medicine* 11(21)

Wong G, Greenhalgh T, Westhorp G, Buckingham J and Pawson R (2013b) RAMESES publication standards: Meta-narrative reviews. *Journal of Advanced Nursing* 69(5): 987–1004

Wong SS, Wilczynski NL and Haynes RB, for the Hedges Team (2004) Developing optimal search strategies for detecting clinically relevant qualitative studies in MEDLINE. *Medinfo* 11(1): 311–16

Zitomer MR and Goodwin D (2014) Gauging the quality of qualitative research in adapted physical activity. *Adapted Physical Activity* 31(3): 193–218

Appendix

Data Extraction form

Name of reviewer:	Date of data extraction:	Study ID:
Nancy	20|8|14	—

Study Details:

Lead Author	Ba
Year	2013
Country (ies)	CHINA.
Start of recruitment	Dec 2008
End of recruitment	Dec 2011
Intended duration of follow up for each patient (months)- please state maximum	
Number of recruiting centres:	? 1
If >1 recruiting centres, is the trial cluster randomised?	Yes / No / (NA)
Type of report: (F=full text; A=abstract; U=unpublished)	F
Language	english .
What is the study evaluating? (A= pleurodesis agent; B= mode of admin of pleurodesis; C= other method to optimise pleurodesis; D = IPC)	C

Eligibility Checklist:

INCLUSION CRITERIA	Answer to all must be yes
Is the study population >16 years of age?	✓
Does the study population have symptomatic pleural effusion from an underlying malignant process?	✓
Is the trial an RCT or randomised cross over trial?	✓

EXCLUSION CRITERIA	Answer to all must be no
Does the study include patients with both malignant and non malignant disease, with no clear distinction between the groups in the results section?	No
Is the study evaluating the effect of a drug administered via a method other than the intra-pleural route?	No
Does the study include effusions in a number of different body cavities (eg peritoneum, pericardium), with no distinction between the groups in the results section?	No

Will you continue with data extraction?   (Yes)   No

     If no, please state reason:

Details of the intervention:

Common treatment for all groups (therefore not under comparison)	Drainage of pleural effusion using Hanson trocal.		
Group	**1**	**2**	**3**
Description of intervention	DW - Distilled water 48°C	Physiological saline + cisplatinum	
Dose	500 mls 48°C	500 mls + 70mg cisplat 48°C	
Number of doses given & frequency	① x3 after tube placement ② ICU ③ 2nd + 4th day		
Mode of administration	IP	IP	
Number of patients randomised	12	11	
Number lost to follow up & reasons	O	O	
Which group was used as the control? (tick one)		? ✓	
How did you decide which was the control group? (tick one)	Assumed by data extractor ☑ Stated in paper ☐		

Patient characteristics:

Inclusion criteria	MPE by CXR o CT ≥ 18 yrs Karnofsky preoperated PE 1° canal.
Exclusion criteria	THORACOTOMY LIMITED ENCAPSULATED PE EXTENSIVE PLEURAL ADHESIONS
Type of cancer (A= all; B=meso; C= lung; D=breast/gynae; E=GI; F=urol/renal; G=other (please specify))	A
Other potential confounding variables identified? (eg steroid, NSAIDS, trapped lung, or others.....)	Yes / (No) If yes, please specify:
Were the groups broadly similar at baseline? Eg Age, Sex, WHO PS, Number with trapped lung	Yes / No ? If no, please specify: ALL LISTED TOGETHER.

Study aims:

Relevant primary outcome(s)	Description	How was it measured?	Time point(s) at which it was measured?	Comments
1	C R	UNKNOWN	UNCLEAR.	NOT REALLY EXPLAINED.
2				

Relevant secondary outcome(s)	Description	How was it measured?	Time point(s) at which it was measured?	Comments
1	P.S KARNOFSKY → SCALE	SCALE	AFTER Rx?	
2				
3				
4				
5				
6				
7				
8				
9				

Study Quality (please refer to this when completing the risk of bias table)

Was a power calculation performed?	Yes (No)
Was the study analysed on an intention to treat basis?	Yes / No / (Unsure) BUT ALL INCLUDED
Method of randomisation (eg telephone, envelopes...)	UNKNOWN
Is there substantial missing outcome data? (Eg withdrawals/loss to FU. Are reasons given for withdrawals?)	Yes / (No)/ unsure If yes, please specify:
Were all the aims of the study reported on?	(Yes)/ No / (Unsure)
Any specific points or issues about the study's quality?	VERY POOR REPORTING EVEN WHAT CR IS AND WHEN MEASURED - ? EXCLUDE .

Results: Please insert ABSOLUTE NUMBERS, not %

PLEURODESIS

Timepoint	Group	Pleurodesis success	Pleurodesis failure	Total	Are patients who have died prior to this timepoint included as a success or a failure?*	Method used to define pleurodesis success**
? .	1	10	2	12	NA	? NO FLUID ON X-RAY.
	2	9	2	11	NA	
	3					
	1					
	2					
	3					
	1					
	2					
	3					

* If the data is available, patients who die prior to the timepoint being evaluated should still be included for the analysis (ie if they die with no symptomatic recurrence of effusion, this is a success).
** KEY: A= radiological resolution; B= need for repeat pleural procedure; C= as measured by trial investigators; D= minimal drainage from IPC & radiographic evidence of no significant residual collection; E= other (please specify)

MORTALITY

Timepoint	Group	Number of patients alive	Number of patients dead	Total
	1			
	2			
	3			
	1			
	2			
	3			
	1			
	2			
	3			

MEDIAN SURVIVAL

Group 1				Group 2				Group 3			
n	Median	SD	CI	n	Median	SD	CI	n	Median	SD	CI
12	13m	(30-30m)		11	12.9	4-26m				4-26m	

SYMPTOM SCALE -Please include quality of life, pain and breathlessness scales or any other symptom scores. If reported, please also include any score of patient acceptability of the intervention.

1. Which scale? _KARNOFFSKY_ .

Time point	Group	Baseline				Follow up				Change			
		n	Mean	SD	CI	n	Mean	SD	CI	n	Mean	SD	CI
?	1	12	54	?+40%	12	77.2	?		12	23.2		
	2	11	54.4	?	11	77.5	?		11	23.1		
	3												
	1												
	2												
	3												
	1												
	2												
	3												

2. Which scale? _____

Time point	Group	Baseline				Follow up				Change			
		n	Mean	SD	CI	n	Mean	SD	CI	n	Mean	SD	CI
	1												
	2												
	3												
	1												
	2												
	3												
	1												
	2												
	3												

3. Which scale? _____

Time point	Group	Baseline				Follow up				Change			
		n	Mean	SD	CI	n	Mean	SD	CI	n	Mean	SD	CI
	1												
	2												
	3												
	1												
	2												
	3												
	1												
	2												
	3												

4. Which scale? _____

Time point	Group	Baseline				Follow up				Change			
		n	Mean	SD	CI	n	Mean	SD	CI	n	Mean	SD	CI
	1												
	2												
	3												
	1												
	2												
	3												
	1												
	2												
	3												

DURATION OF INPATIENT STAY (if available)

Timepoint	Group	n	Mean	SD	95% CI
Randomisation to discharge	1				
	2				
	3				
	1				
	2				
	3				

COSTS (if available)

Timepoint	Group	n	Mean	SD	95% CI
	1				
	2				
	3				
	1				
	2				
	3				

ADVERSE EVENTS/ COMPLICATIONS FROM THE INTERVENTION:

Event	Group	Number effected	Number not effected	Total	Comments
	1	SAID NO AE			
	2				
	3				
	1				
	2				
	3				
	1				
	2				
	3				
	1				
	2				
	3				

Risk of bias tool:

Domain	Description and support for judgement (PLEASE FILL THIS IN!!!)	Review authors judgment HIGH= High risk of bias LOW= low risk of bias
Sequence generation - Low risk of bias (any truly random process, eg random number table; computer generated) - High risk of bias (any non-random process, eg odd or even DOB; hospital or clinic record number) - Unclear risk of bias: the trial may or may not be free of bias	NOT STATED	Was the allocation sequence adequately generated? (HIGH) / LOW / (UNCLEAR)
Allocation concealment Could the allocation could have been foreseen prior to or during recruitment? - Low risk of bias (e.g. telephone or central randomisation; consecutively numbered sealed opaque envelopes) - High risk of bias (open random allocation; unsealed or non-opaque envelopes, alternation; date of birth) - Unclear risk of bias- the trial may or may not be free of bias	NOT ENOUGH INFO	Was allocation adequately concealed? HIGH / LOW / (UNCLEAR)
Blinding of participants, personnel and outcome assessors - Low risk of bias: Blinded and method used for blinding described - Unknown risk: if they stated that they were blinded, but did not describe how it was achieved. - High risk of bias: Unblinded	NONE STATED.	Was knowledge of the allocated intervention adequately prevented during the study? HIGH / LOW / (UNCLEAR)
Incomplete outcome data - Include whether study analysed on an intention to treat basis - Is these lots of missing outcome data? (Eg withdrawls/ loss to FU. Are reasons given for withdrawls?)	ALL THERE	Were incomplete outcome data adequately addressed? HIGH / (LOW) / UNCLEAR
Selective outcome reporting - Low risk of bias: all outcomes pre-defined and reported, or all clinically relevant and expected outcomes were reported. - Uncertain risk: Unclear whether all pre-defined and clinically relevant were reported. - High risk of bias: one or more clinically relevant and reasonably expected outcomes were not reported, and data on these outcomes were likely to have been recorded.	ALL THERE	Are reports of the study free of suggestion of selective outcome reporting? HIGH / (LOW) / UNCLEAR
Other sources of bias - Low risk of bias: the trial appears to be free of other bias, eg industry bias, academic bias) - Uncertain risk of bias: Unclear if other sources of bias - High risk of bias: Other factors in that could put trial at risk of bias (for example, for-profit involvement, authors have conducted trials on the same topic). ** Also comment here on • method used to define pleurodesis • inc/exc patients with trapped lung	NO DEFINITION OF OUTCOME - CR NO TIMINGS? NO RANDOMISATION METHOD ? EXCLUDE	Was the study apparently free of other problems that could put it at a high risk of bias? (HIGH) / LOW / UNCLEAR

Index